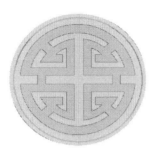

Achieving Fulfillment & Prosperity

Young Adult Edition

by C.C. Talley

www.achievingfulfillment.com

WELCOME

Thank you for purchasing this book!

There is one thing that we all have in common. We were born into a world of opportunity. It usually takes growing up to see it.

Each of us grew up in different childhood home environments. Some in poverty, some from privilege. Some with the freedom to roam like a band of pirates, some in controlled captivity with no regard for innocence. Some built playhouses, some built forts. Some worked in the garden, some worked on chores. Some chased fireflies, some chased the bus. Some rode bikes all day with wild abandonment, some rode on the back of their bulldog while he chased rocks around the yard. Some played baseball in old dirt fields, some played video games. Some cooked with grandma, some fished with grandpa. Most of us danced, sang and wished on shooting stars.
No matter what kind of childhood you had, ultimately, you learned a lot of hard lessons during those years.

That world eventually came to a stop and the world of confusion and responsibility came crashing down on us all. Some of us just make it through high school while others go on to college.

I'm sure you are asking the same old question that we all ask. Where is this crazy ride going to take me?

You may be a young adult in need of life skills and practical training, a young professional preparing for a big career, in between jobs looking for the next opportunity or wanting to become the best version of yourself and need some help developing a plan of action.

The information in this book will offer you guidance and foresight to start your life journey towards fulfillment and prosperity. A lot of the content is advice that I wish I received at an earlier age. Some of the suggestions will take a lot of work but trust that they will lead to a positive result.

If you enjoy the book, please to recommend it to everyone in your circle of influence.

My hope is that you take away a few notes of inspiration and challenge from this book. Use it as a compass or road map for your travels.

My desire is for you to succeed wildly beyond your expectations.

Before you start reading, please take a few deep breaths and slow exhales to center your mind. Say a few words of thanks for the things you are grateful for today.

1. INTRODUCTION

Life is an ocean of choices. Navigate wisely through the storms and you will enjoy the destinations more abundantly and with complete fulfillment.
-C.C. Talley

Our culture likes to use words like rich, popular, genius, Gucci, fleek, GOAT. These terms are more humorous than anything. If you want a good laugh, try to explain them to grandparents that still believe in the notion of chivalry and proper dialect. As entertaining as they are, these titles are not always healthy or sustainable. Let's introduce and define two words that our culture does not use enough. Let's place them at the top of our shared vocabulary and goals.

Fulfillment = achievement, gratification, contentment, attainment, perfection, realization. It is the natural consequence of doing the right thing. It is not pleasure. It is happiness.

Prosperity = accomplishment, benefit, growth, wealth, well-being

These two words are understood to be a result or product of something. That something is life. Our existence is reliant on so many things: air, water, food, sleep and shelter are our basic needs. Once these physiological and safety needs are met, we are provided an opportunity for growth and change.

Self-actualization
desire to become the most that one can be

Esteem
respect, self-esteem, status, recognition, strength, freedom

Love and belonging
friendship, intimacy, family, sense of connection

Safety needs
personal security, employment, resources, health, property

Physiological needs
air, water, food, shelter, sleep, clothing, reproduction

Abraham Maslow spent countless years researching what he defined as Maslow's Hierarchy of Needs which explains the next levels of behavioral motivation: love and belonging, esteem and self-actualization. These levels involve achieving a state of being called happiness. How in the world do we do that? How do we attain happiness? Bobby McFerrin made millions of dollars from his song 'Don't Worry Be Happy'! Maybe he knows the answer? Could there be a magic switch behind our bed to flip every morning? Do our bathroom mirrors have the power to instantly transform us from being mad or grumpy, to happy?

Here is a complex but agile solution involving another idea that we should add to our shared vocabulary and goals: balance through personal development.

Balance = harmony, equity, parity, symmetry

Why is balance important?

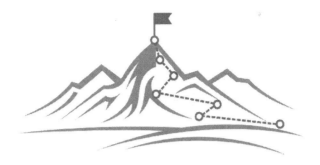

The most used analogy for success is the 'mountain climb'. As we study this and apply it to our own lives, the takeaways are as follows:
1. Educate ourselves on the terrain so that we might chart the path of least resistance.
2. Train our bodies so that we are able to endure the journey. In other words, let us neither fall backwards to the base nor forward on our face! There lies the focus on balance. Think about any object that stands upright. In order to remain in that state, it must be balanced.

Here is a new cultural word for the urban dictionary { PALI } = [paa-lee] a blend of balance and harmony. Buddhist's use this word (Tatramajjhattatā) and define it as a mental attitude of balance and neutrality of mind.

Life Balance requires a solid foundation built upon wise decisions and purposeful development. The next three chapters will dive into the main areas of our life that must be focused on first in order to achieve a successful balance. The following chapters will address physical, mental and emotional states of being.

(Physical Health + Mental Health + Emotional Health)
Balance

= Optimal Health and Self-Awareness

Once we have reached our state of optimal health and self-awareness, we are then able to give our best to our families, partners, friends, companies, community and world. In return, we will find true happiness.

We each have our own journey. There is no darkness that cannot be overcome. There are no failures that will keep us down indefinitely. There are only opportunities to learn and grow. Make good choices.

2. PHYSICAL BALANCE

Physical health is vital for our overall well-being. Well-being can be described as free from illness or injury, controlling optimal weight, producing sustainable energy, having clean personal hygiene, good dental health and sufficient sleep. Here are 4 keys to wellbeing:

1. Good Nutrition
2. Regular Physical Activity
3. Bathing and Cleaning
4. Adequate Rest

There is a link between our belly and our brain. Neurotransmitters create chemicals that activate bodily sensations. These sensations produce feelings of happiness, energy and excitement, or stress and anxiety. They control the way we think and behave. Most of them are produced in our gut. Also produced in our intestines are serotonin, nature's antidepressant. Only 10% of serotonin is produced in our brain. The right balance of microbes can help prevent and treat disease. If you are questioning this, answer these questions - Has stress ever caused you stomach issues? Have you ever had butterfly feelings in your belly?

Good nutrition simply comes from eating right!
It doesn't have to be complicated. As in all other areas of our lives, we need to develop a plan.

Start by determining which foods items you would like to cut out of your diet. Take small steps by shifting just a few weekly food and beverage choices. How often do you eat candy, chips, bread, and heavy or fried foods? What about soda or energy drinks? These things lead to disease, pain, functional complications and often shorter life spans. We can reduce the risk of high blood pressure, heart disease and stroke by eating less sodium. Sugar is the worst thing we can ingest. It has no positive effect on our bodies but does cause obesity and diabetes. We should also avoid foods that cause inflammation. We need to eat real-whole-clean food!

One fun challenge that will promote a natural diet is to grow your own food. If you have a porch or even a sidewalk, you can grow your own raised garden beds. EMSCO makes one that has casters and a watering system. Some of the best compost can be made from coffee grounds, egg shells, vegetable scraps, banana peels and grass clippings in a 5-gallon bucket. For the best results, seal the bucket and let it sit through a hot summer. Mix this with a little soil and you have an all-natural, rocket-fueled garden fertilizer. Many farmers markets have seedlings that can jump start your project. If you have time, buy organic seeds online and study your growing zone to figure out what grows best in your area and when to plant.

Eat in moderation! It is very important to eat breakfast, lunch and dinner with a few snacks in between. Breakfast gives us the energy that we need to Rock the Day! Please do not misunderstand this to mean that we should order the Grandma's Kitchen Sink Sampler at Pancake House every day. If you do not have time to cook your own food, be smart in your decisions when you eat out. If fast food is the only option, do a little research on what the most delicious and healthy options are on the menu. "Eat This Not That!" has a good guide to help you make some of those decisions.

In general, health care professionals recommend that women might eat 300 to 500 calories at each meal and that men should consume 400 to 600 calories at breakfast, lunch, and dinner, and then enjoy two to three 150-calorie snacks during the day. Fruit and nuts are a great snacking option. Many trainers suggest finding a 'real food' protein bar that you enjoy eating like RXBAR. Of course, all of this depends on our weight, age, sex and physical activity. Here is a sample of estimated calorie needs per day:

MALES				FEMALES			
Age	Sedentary	Moderately Active	Active	Age	Sedentary	Moderately Active	Active
18	2,400	2,800	3,200	18	1,800	2,000	2,400
19-20	2,600	2,800	3,000	19-20	2,000	2,200	2,400
21-25	2,400	2,800	3,000	21-25	2,000	2,200	2,400
26-30	2,400	2,600	3,000	26-30	1,800	2,000	2,400
31-35	2,400	2,600	3,000	31-35	1,800	2,000	2,200
36-40	2,400	2,600	2,800	36-40	1,800	2,000	2,200

Sedentary means a lifestyle that includes only the physical activity of independent living.

Moderately Active means a lifestyle that includes physical activity equivalent to walking about 1.5 to 3 miles per day at 3 to 4 miles per hour, in addition to the activities of independent living.

Active means a lifestyle that includes physical activity equivalent to walking more than 3 miles per day at 3 to 4 miles per hour, in addition to the activities of independent living.

Estimates for females do not include women who are pregnant or breastfeeding.

Stay hydrated! Find a water bottle that is easy to tote around and holds at least 16oz. Be sure to fill it up 4 times throughout the day. Or you could invest in a 32oz bottle with markings from Cactaki and fill it up twice each day. Health authorities commonly recommend that we ingest 8 x 8-ounce glasses of water, which equals about 2 liters, or half a gallon. Without enough water, your body cannot function properly.

How do we get rid of fat? The average fat molecule makeup is $C_{55}H_{104}O_6$
Your body has to turn fat molecules into triglycerides and then they are released as carbon dioxide and water. Here is the secret: Eat Less + Move More + Keep Breathing

What about Fad Diets? There are many options of diets for weight loss. One popular diet right now is the Keto diet. Ketogenesis is when you starve your body of carbohydrates (high protein and fat diet), but may be linked to depression. If you are considering one, first ask your doctor to confirm that your body will be receptive to the effort and that you will not have negative side effects. Also make sure that the diet you're considering is not sponsored by Gordos Cheese Dip!

Exercise Daily!
First, we need to identify what is most important to you today? Do you want to lose a sizeable amount of weight, get toned, gain muscle mass or just drop a few pounds? Next you need to find a fitness routine that works best for your schedule. You don't have to have a lot of money to accomplish your goals. You don't even have to have a gym membership. You can watch a workout on YouTube in your room, go to a community fitness center, attend a Yoga class, Crossfit, run, bike, swim, walk or hike. You don't even have to use weights. Bodyweight workouts can produce big results. Herschel Walker, one of the greatest athletes ever only used bodyweight workouts. TRX all-in-one training systems are a great option for anyone that wants to get a full workout in your garage but doesn't want to pay a lot of money or buy a bunch of bulky equipment.

Start your day by stretching for a few minutes. Stretching prepares muscles for performance and reduces injury. There are a few stretching video links at the end of this book. Be sure to check them out.

If you need some inspiration, start a workout playlist of your favorite 'upbeat' songs. If you do not currently have a routine, grab your headphones or AirPods and head out the door for a jog. We should all make cardiovascular exercise a weekly priority. An elevated heart rate and sweat are the keys to burning fat and creating higher energy levels. There are a few cardio workout links at the end of the book that you may enjoy. The intensity of group workouts tends to promote bigger results than going solo. Sign up for a class and join the movement!

Keeping fit is one of the most challenging parts of our lives. Especially as we get older. We must commit to the long run. Getting in shape or losing weight takes time. Be consistent with your routine.

Let's set some Goals. Start by making a list of activities that you would like to achieve.

Here are a few examples:
>Exercise 5 days each week
>Lower your body fat percentage by 1%
>Master a skill
>Train for an event
>Run a 5k
>Lose 2 pounds in 3 weeks

Get enough sleep!
Young adults need 7 - 9 hours of sleep. Try your best to create a routine for your week that remains consistent. If you are having trouble sleeping, go see your doctor. Insomnia, restless leg syndrome, jetlag, anxiety, depression and certain medications could be the cause of your restless nights.

Breathe!
Take slow, intentional, deep breaths throughout the day. There are a few breathing apps that may help you with this. Set reminders on your phone if you have to. Breathing exercises can also help reduce anxiety and stress.

What are your current challenges?
Identify your top 3 unhealthy habits and create a plan to overcome the source.

Bad Habit #1:
Source:

Bad Habit #2:
Source:

Bad Habit #3:
Source:

Fill in the blank after these sentences:
I can make my number one bad habit hard to keep doing
by_____

I can make my number one goal easy to achieve
by_____

Diet and Fitness Plan
Here is a spreadsheet to get you started. Be sure to log onto
www.achievingfulfillment.com/book-tools Click the link to the
Google Sheet version. Save your own copy first and then you
will be able to edit it for your own development plan. There are
a few recipes below the spreadsheet. The document is
formatted to pull any workout or recipe into your 'Select One'
dropdown menu.

DATE:	MONDAY	TUESDAY	WEDNESDAY	THURSDAY	FRIDAY	SATURDAY	SUNDAY
BREAKFAST	Select One	Select One	Select One	Select One	Select One	Select One	Select One
LUNCH	Select One	Select One	Select One	Select One	Select One	Select One	Select One
SNACKS	Select One	Select One	Select One	Select One	Select One	Select One	Select One
DINNER	Select One	Select One	Select One	Select One	Select One	Select One	Select One
Workout	Select One	Select One	Select One	Select One	Select One	Select One	Select One

Something's just not right!

If you are feeling like something inside is just not right, have a nutritionist give you an assessment to determine if you have a deficiency and a gastroenterologist give you a check for a hereditary illness or other condition. Bottom line is if you have any pain or discomfort, go see a doctor.

Avoid Self Destructive Temptations of Substance Abuse!

Illegal and legally abused substances offer nothing but a quick generic cerebral release from reality that only stunts our potential for growth. They hinder our purpose and in time or if consumed in abundance will ultimately kill us. They will rob us of self-worth, purpose and confidence. Many people struggle with addiction. Addiction dislocates people from social life and creates an individualized world of self-absorption and destructive behaviors. Drug addiction can create a time known as 'The Lost Years' where there is no productivity or advancement; only victimization and deterioration of the mind and body. There is no joy in this journey. Only heartbreak!

Top Performers - ask Jillian Michaels, Dwayne (The Rock) Johnson, Chris Hemsworth, Beyoncé, Madonna or Mark Wahlberg what their daily habits are? They made the commitment to work as hard as they can, in order to give the world their best.
Make this statement every morning: 'I'm getting better at getting better!'

Accountability Partner (AP)
We all need an accountability partner. This is a necessary step for growth. Find someone that you trust will not judge you. The relationship should be a partnership. They must agree to support you in your development and not discourage you. It probably does not need to be your best friend. They need to be able to push you in times of doubt. If you can afford the cost, get together with a personal trainer.

New healthy habits will lead to a life filled with rich physical enjoyment. Once you determine the best plan for development, commit to working on it every day until it becomes a behavior that you cannot live without. New habits can take many months to become an installed development.

Now that you are focusing on being active, you also must make time to relax. Your body needs recovery. Massage therapists or a good soak in the tub can help ease your tension. There are other forms of therapy that you may find enjoyable. Check into Tai Chi, meditation, Yoga, music and art therapy, aromatherapy or hydrotherapy.

Live healthy and stay balanced!

NTAL BALANCE

al Intelligence is defined as brain activity that addresses perception, learning, memory, reasoning and problem solving. Education is one of the biggest contributors to our growth. This is also known as IQ.

As infants, our brain was influenced by interaction with our parents and caregivers. The brain is designed for continual growth and learning.

How do we keep our brains healthy? Feed Them! A healthy brain is an active brain. Be intellectually curious. Read as much as possible. Always seek more knowledge.

"Live as if you were to die tomorrow. Learn as if you were to live forever."
-Mahatma Gandi

Positive Influence is critical to setting your mental compass. There are many global and local issues that are not easy to understand. Your value as a contributing citizen to society can be increased with each subject that on which you become educated. You do not have to become an expert on every topic, but a good goal is to understand enough about the ones that interest you that you can carry on a conversation without sounding completely ignorant. Here are a few topics you might want to research:

Real Estate
Foreign Language
Household Repairs
Automobile Maintenance
Cooking
Nutrition
First Aid
Social Etiquette
Insurance
Negotiating

Social Media Safety
Survival Skills
Local Government
Taxes
Global Environmental Issues
World Religions
Micro and Macro Economics
Check out some inspiring and mind-bending books from these
authors: Malcom Gladwell, Tony Robbins, Brendon Burchard,
Eric Thomas, and Warren Buffett.

Students

Your 'time' is the most valuable thing that you have right now.
Use it wisely.

Ask for what you need. Pride has a tendency to get in our way. If
you need assistance with school or life events, please ask for it.

Honor your teachers and professors. They are experts in their
field, sacrificing much to be in their positions. Get to know
them. You might be surprised to hear the stories of their
journey.

Just Two Questions

One night four college kids stayed out late partying and having a
good time. They paid no mind to the test they had scheduled for
the next day and didn't study. In the morning, they hatched a
plan to get out of taking their test. They covered themselves
with grease and dirt and went to the Dean's office. Once there,
they said they had been to a wedding the previous night and on
the way back they got a flat tire and had to push the car back to
campus.
The Dean listened to their tale of woe and thought. He offered
them a retest three days later. They thanked him and accepted
his offer.
When the test day arrived, they went to the Dean. The Dean put
them all in separate rooms for the test. They were fine with this
since they had all studied hard. Then they saw the test. It had
two questions.

1) Your Name _____ (1 Points)
2) Which tire burst? _____ (99 Points)
Options – (a) Front Left (b) Front Right (c) Back Left (d) Back Right
The lesson: always be responsible and make wise decisions.

Source: (https://www.livin3.com/5-motivational-and-inspiring-short-stories)

Learning / Studying Tips
We all have different learning styles. Some people are multi-sensory learners that use a combination of techniques. Here are some tips for each style:

Visual Learners
Clues = strong sense of color, needs to see it to know it, difficulty with spoken directions, overreaction to sounds, trouble following lectures, misinterpretation of words, may have artistic ability.
Learning Tips = write out directions, use graphics to reinforce learning, color coding to organize notes, use flow charts/illustrations/diagrams for note taking.

Auditory Learners (oral / interactive)
Clues = difficulty following written directions, difficulty with reading, problems with writing, prefers to get information by listening, needs to hear it to know it, inability to read body language and facial expressions.
Learning Tips = have test questions or directions read aloud or recorded, record class notes and lectures, learn by interviewing or participating in discussions.

Kinesthetic Learners (physical / tactile)
Clues = prefers hands on learning, difficulty sitting still, can assemble parts without reading directions, learns better when physical activity is involved, may be very well coordinated or athletic.
Learning Tips = frequent breaks in study periods, experiential learning (lab work, role playing, building models), memorize or practice while walking or exercising.

Test Taking Tips
Don't cram before the exam! Pulling off an all-nighter simply doesn't work. Your brain needs time to digest the information. The best way to learn is to study the same information in redundancy over a period of days. Create a study schedule in 20 to 30-minute bursts. Do something relaxing the day before and get a good night's rest. Avoid caffeine and sugar. Before entering the exam, take 5 minutes to focus on your breathing and calm your nerves. Tell yourself, "I'm going to Ace It!" Believe in yourself and trust the preparation that you put into the subject.

If you are struggling to comprehend a subject or do not find it interesting, find a tutor or mentor. Ask them to help you make the content 'applicable' to your life. For example, if you are studying about a profit and loss statement in accounting, but are having difficulty making sense of it, find someone that uses the report in a real-life setting. Introduce yourself to a local restaurant general manager and ask if they can walk you through one of theirs. Twenty minutes of their time can help you understand the tangible relationship between the costs involved in operating the business and the bottom line of profit. Just offer to buy them breakfast!

Higher Education / Trade School / Mentorship
High school female brains are more developed than male brains and typically can gauge what their next step in life is. If you don't know if college is right for you, get a job and work until you find the right path. Research your degree. Don't enroll just to 'Go to College'. Community colleges offer a lot of flexibility with two-year programs. FedEx has a fully funded college plan for qualified candidates seeking a finance degree. Trade schools are industry specific and are a solid choice for anyone entertaining a career in one of their many fields. Not everyone will have the ability to attend college or higher learning. There are plenty of other options. Thomas Edison only had 3 months of formal schooling in his entire life. He went to the college of Learning By Doing. If you do not have the financial capacity to continue higher education, work and save money until you can

afford it. Find a mentor. For example, if you plan on driving for a ride sharing company (Uber or Lyft), find another driver that is making good money doing it and ask them to mentor you. Learn their secret hot spots and the best times to work. If you really want to go on an adventure, enlist in the military. In exchange for your time and dedication, you can learn a new skill, receive a free education, travel and receive veteran benefits.

As Gaming Becomes More Prominent
If you play video games, limit your gaming to 30 minutes a day. Halo, Call of Duty and Super Mario will not help you grow. In fact, excessive gaming may stall or even stunt your potential if you become so fixated on them that you don't leave your room. There is a community of professional gamers that do make a good living, but don't be fooled. These professionals train like athletes and most of maintain focus on a balanced life.

Creating healthy habits as a young adult will transfer to your later years. Have you ever noticed that aging seems to speed up when people retire? Especially when retirees do not socialize or use their mind. Many States offer free college courses for adults over the age of 65. Why do you think States made that an option? To promote mental activity and an opportunity to achieve additional life goals. Feed your brain!

4. EMOTIONAL BALANCE

Emotional EQ is identifiably different than IQ. We cannot predict someone's emotional intelligence based on how smart they are. Think of it as street smarts or situational awareness. Our mental strength can be developed and refined the same as training in any other area of our lives. This subject may sound like a bunch of psychological mumbo jumbo gumbo, but we must understand how our minds work and how we can control them, even more than our physique.

Mental Strength is brain activity that addresses the thoughts and behaviors that affect the overall quality of our lives. This involves developing daily habits that build mental muscle. It also involves giving up bad habits that hold us back.

1. Regulating your thoughts - Regulating your thoughts involves learning how to train your brain to think in a helpful manner. That may mean ignoring self-doubt or replacing self-criticism with self-compassion.
2. Managing your emotions - Being aware of your emotions allows you to understand how those feelings influence the way you think and behave. It may involve embracing emotions even when they are uncomfortable. Or it may be about acting contrary to your emotions, when those feelings don't serve you well.
3. Behaving productively - Choosing to take action that will improve your life is key to becoming mentally strong. Especially when you struggle with motivation or delayed gratification. (Morin 2017)

Emotional Intelligence is scientifically described as the gap between a stimulus and response. Let's think of it as our ability to understand the emotions that we are having and how we respond to them. It's the connection between our emotional brain (limbic system) and our rational brain.

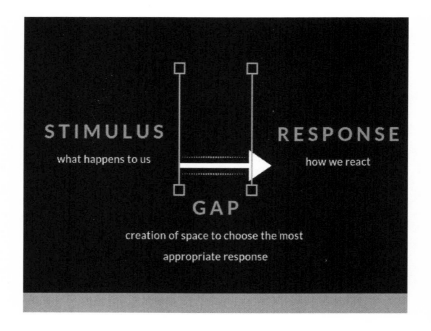

The gap is either a pause before a decision is made or an immediate reaction made without thought. Here is an example of poor emotional intelligence: if you think money will provide an opportunity for you to have more balance and make better decisions, look up the fines imposed on professional athletes. It is astonishing - personal fouls, ejections, inappropriate language and gestures, conduct detrimental to the team, fighting, illegal drug use, dui, and the list goes on. Can you imagine forfeiting over $6,000,000 due to your own lack of emotional intelligence? https://www.casino.org/biggest-sports-fines/

Areas of EI

1. Self Awareness - The ability to accurately perceive your emotions and drives, as well as their effect on others.
2. Internal Motivation - A passion to work that goes beyond money and status, such as inner vision of what is important in life or the joy of doing something.

3. Self-Regulation - The ability to redirect disruptive impulses and moods. The ability to think before acting.
4. Empathy - The ability to understand the emotional makeup or feelings of other people and the willingness to treat them according to their emotional reactions.
5. Social Competence - The ability to accurately pick up on the emotions of other people or the awareness of others. Social skills include proficiency in managing relationships and an ability to build rapport with others by finding common ground. Have you ever walked into a room and 'felt the mood'?

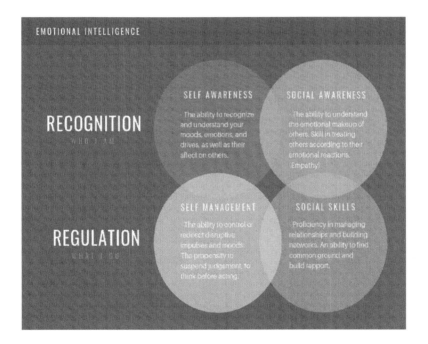

There are many young adult life situations that require a high level of EQ.

Starting the day:
Begin your morning with positive thoughts. Have you heard of the 'power of attitude'? The merit of this subject should not be

taken lightly. If you are unable to control your own negative emotions before you eat breakfast, you will be attempting to push your mental car around all day instead of drive it, because you neglected to fill up the tank. Top your mind off with thoughts of success, love, compassion, gratitude and drive.

Responding to a situation that causes any level of anxiety or discomfort:
Instead of quickly reacting to a confrontational situation, take time to process what is going on. This takes patience and practice. Start by asking yourself a few questions. What is causing the negative emotion? What is the motive of the person communicating with you? Sometimes the best words to respond with are, "thank you for bringing this to my attention, if it's OK with you, I'm going to take some time to find the best solution and get back with you". The truth is that most people you feel are attacking you are actually frustrated because they don't have the information that they need or are trying to blame someone else for their own mistakes. During a heated confrontation, take six seconds to slow down the flood of chemicals that are being produced and weight the benefits or costs of your actions. This process will allow you to view the situation through a conditional lens instead of a wide-angle lens. Every situation is different and when you treat each interaction as such, you will make better decisions versus if you are quick to anger and treat each person with the same disrespectful response. If you receive a text or email that makes your head hot and increases your heart rate, take 5 minutes to reflect on the most appropriate response.

Tapping into Daily Drive:
This requires the ability to maintain focus and determination to achieve a goal despite the difficulty. There will be days when you are tired, sick or deflated, but you must fight through the challenges. Haters are always going to hate. Just make sure that you do not buy a ticket to their show! You have your own performance to work on.

Develop 'Ultimate Confidence'

Ultimate confidence is the capacity to control personal judgement, ability and power. You must believe in yourself. Self-doubt is paralyzing. There should be a class in high school titled Mastery of Confidence. Since this class is not available, we are left to figure it out together. You are not alone. We are a community of supporters and believers in you. There will always be someone that has an argument or negative comment. Get away from the people that tear you down. The key to unbreakable self-confidence is daily declaration. Let's develop your ultimate confidence statement.

What are your top 3 most appreciated personal attributes or strengths?
1.

2.

3.

What are your top 3 goals?
1.

2.

3.

Great! Now let's construct your ultimate confidence statement. Marry the two lists and repeat them 3 times every day. Here is an example: "I am healthy, I am happy, I serve others, I am successful, I am debt free, I am loved." Continue to shape these statements as you grow. Maybe one day you will only have two statements: "I am fulfilled", "I change lives".

Courage is the mental fortitude to overcome fear or pain in the hope of achieving a goal or fighting illness. Let's get one thing straight here - You cannot live a life of courage without disappointing some people. If you are making intentional decisions that reflect authentic motivation, then you are serving yourself first. Do not let this idea dissuade you. You were not created to please only your parents or teachers. You already have the courage inside you. Call it out!

Emotional Intelligence is all about controlling your thoughts and behaviors. Here is a list of low emotional intelligence versus high emotional intelligence.

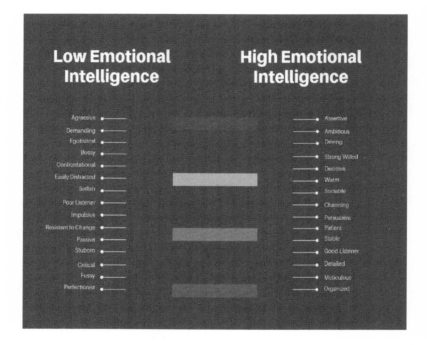

Emotional Intelligence is the foundation for the critical skills of success. The top skills that we should focus on are decision making, time management, communication, team work, social skills, anger management, flexibility, accountability, assertiveness, trust, customer service, presentation skills, empathy, change tolerance and stress tolerance.

Top 3 keys to increasing EQ:

1. Get your stress under control. Stress compromises your immune system. It is also linked to heart disease, depression and obesity.

2. Get the right amount of sleep. When we sleep, neurons clean up toxic proteins. Avoid taking sleeping aids, they prohibit the neurons from working.

3. Get caffeine intake under control. Avoid drinking it late at night.

"Remember that stress doesn't come from what's going on in your life. It comes from your thoughts about what's going on in your life."
– Andrew J. Bernstein

You have more than likely experienced some type of burn out before while preparing for a test or attempting to finish a big project at work.

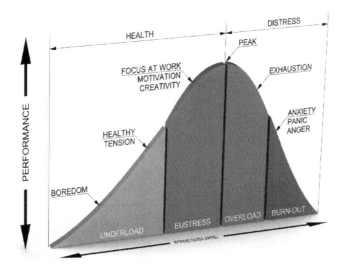

When you start to feel stressed, cultivate an attitude of gratitude! Studies at UC Berkeley found that it psychologically lowered the levels of cortisol. Cortisol is the main hormone involved in stress and the fight-or-flight response. This is a natural and protective response to a perceived threat or danger. Increased levels of cortisol can result in a rapid heart rate, dry mouth, upset stomach and panic.

Fear Paralyzes Growth and Development
The first step to controlling anxiety is to clearly understand what your triggers are. Everyone has certain buttons that when pushed, send us into meltdown mode. It could be a confrontational person that approaches you in anger. It might be the feeling of running late for a meeting. Sometimes it is the critic that is tearing your work apart due to their own undigested pain. The second step to controlling anxiety is to acknowledge that anxiety comes from our own fears. The fear of failure. The fear of being late. The fear of disappointing others. The fear of being hurt. Fear is not a big evil force lurking in the night. It is a psychological emotion that lives and dies between your two ears. If allowed to breathe, fear can produce "self-doubt, insecurity, lack of confidence, shyness, inhibition or timidity (a reluctance to be assertive, express, or even be yourself). Whatever form fear takes, your willingness to face it squarely will determine your fate in the high country of human potential. The most constructive way to influence your emotions is to do something." (Millman, 1998)

We have two primary emotions; Love and Fear. Choose Love.

Mental Illness
Mental Illness is a disorder that negatively affects your mood, thinking and behavior. The biggest are depression, anxiety, schizophrenia and eating disorders. They typically stem from isolation or loneliness. When a person cuts off connection with society, the brain does not receive the stimulus that is required to fully produce a balance of chemicals. The chemical imbalance

sometimes tricks the mind into thinking that solitude is good. It is not. Mental illness robs the mind of energy, passion, love and kindness. The sickness turns a mind into a fearful mess of confusion and anger. Mental illness has links to physical illness, homelessness and mass killings.

"Mental health among young adults is an area of grave concern in today's world. Early adulthood is a time of heightened psychological vulnerability and onset of serious mental health disorders, a problem compounded by failure to recognize illness or to seek treatment. Along with substance use, mental health disorders are the greatest source of disability among young adults in the United States." (Bonnie,Sepulveda, 2014)

The suicide and mass killing epidemic is often not a parenting issue but lack of education by our society and lack of focus on mental illness. Once something evil like this finds its way into our culture, we have to make it part of our educational system. We must talk to our children and each other. As young adults, we need to be the leaders. Make a stand for mental health.

Not all wounds are visible. We all need help! We all need each other! There is no shame in asking for it.

It is not easy to confront or overcome depression and anxiety! Sometimes medication is necessary. Other times people can fight the illness by finding a new passion, listening to music, journaling, growing a garden, calling an old friend, creating a new business idea, doing breathing exercises, attending a Yoga class, adopting a new pet or going on a trip. If you are going through a tough time in your life, having feelings of depression or even thoughts of suicide, or have been the victim of any physical (bullying), mental or sexual abuse, please visit this website:

https://www.crisistextline.org/

Own Your Influences

Do not be persuaded by people or marketing ploys until you have asked yourself if this person, idea, resource or product is in alignment with my true self. If the answer is 'no but I would look like or sound like them', you could be making a costly mistake. Your time is just as valuable as your money. If you sign up to watch a class on 'How To Give Your Goldfish A Bath' because you like the way the models look in the ad, you are wasting your time. Young adulthood is a wildly adventurous time in our lives. Living on our own requires that we make our own choices, fight our own doubts and find our own joy. Do not rely on others to generate or sustain your happiness. Find it within your own mind and express it with your emotions.

5. PASSION and INSPIRATION

> "I wanna set fear on fire and give dreamin' a fair shot.
> And never give up whether anybody cares or not."
> - 'Gospel' by John Moreland

What are your dreams? What are your passions? What are your goals? What are your skills? What is your purpose?

Let's agree on one rule here: never laugh at anyone's dreams, no matter how big, small or irrational they may seem. The world needs us all. There are professional magicians and fishermen. Someone needs to be the financial analyst, chocolate taster, drycleaner, florist, insurance salesperson, first responder, screenwriter, rapper, dance instructor, golf instructor, lifeguard, record producer, wine maker, bobble-head designer and dancing seahorse at Disney World.

One of the biggest dreams that has become an enterprise is Cirque du Soleil. I can't begin to imagine what dreams Guy Laliberte and Giles Ste-Croix had before they met to found the traveling entertainment company. Another amazing story of super soul dreams, hope and determination is the life of Oprah Winfrey. I wish we could all get 10 minutes of her time to gain wise perspective and inspiration. How about the journey of Elon Musk? That guy has an imagination that is hard to process. His two primary companies, Tesla and SpaceX have become household names like Uber and Google.

What do you love to do or have a high level of interest in? How about cooking, painting, writing, designing, playing sports, creating apps, farming, writing code, speaking, teaching, building, playing or performing music, singing, serving your country in the military, taking pictures, traveling, acting, serving the homeless, aiding with elderly care, law enforcement, inventing, selling, driving a truck, racing a car, flying a plane, training fitness, leading a team, running a company? I don't think anyone has ever been a professional bubble-wrap-popper, but hey, if that's your thing, go for it!

Young adulthood is a propitious time to sample a diversity of experiences. Do not worry about gaining approval from others. Let the inspiration come from within your own heart.

There are countless options but you have limited time. Focus your vision to a list of no more than four areas of interest and be honorably realistic. It's OK if you can only think of one at this moment. There may be extreme talent lying deep inside that you have not discovered yet. You do not have to be a 'creative' person for this focus to work for you. Write down your list:

My Passions:

1.

2.

3.

4.

Now ask yourself the following questions for each of your answers:
1. Can I make a living by pursuing a professional career with my passion or talent?
2. Is it a sustainable career?
3. Has anyone ever accomplished this?
4. Is it possible for me to find mentors that may offer advice?

For your passions, if you answered yes or maybe to all 4 questions, then you may have discovered your purpose. Historically, we do not uncover our true purpose until later in life, but if you feel a passionate calling at a young age, go forth!

Please send us an email with the following items to:
achievingfulfillment@gmail.com
Subject: (Your State and City) / Passions
Content: Your Name / Your Age / Your Passion List

We may be able to help find some resources for you or schedule a meeting next time we swing through your town.

If you do not currently have any passions, don't worry. They will develop over time. Our interests evolve as we gain wisdom and experience.

Now comes the hard part; take the first step. What is standing in the way of your success? What are your obstacles? Money? Time? Lack of support? Don't have the tools or technology? Do you feel threatened, intimidated or judged? Are you downright fearful? Your biggest obstacle is will be excuses. Everybody has them. Excuses don't pay bills or burn calories. Don't give in. Passion comes from an uncontrollable emotion of inspiration. It is a fire burning inside your soul. Once you light the fire, just fan the flame as hard as you can. MAKE IT A RAGING FIRE! This might become your contribution to world.

Focus on your goals and passions every day. There was a book written in 1937 by Napoleon Hill titled 'Think And Grow Rich'. Mr. Hill was able to spend time with some of the biggest movers and shakers of the time, most notably Andrew Carnegie, to analyze the methods of their success. One of the big discoveries was the Law of Attraction! The basic principle is that if you think and focus on attracting something long enough, you will eventually receive it. Think about your desire to live a healthy, joyful and prosperous life and choose what you want to manifest. Practice daily affirmations and visualizations. Picture yourself already having these blessings. Disconnect yourself from a brand or actual product. The law of attraction states that positive or negative thoughts will manifest themselves in reality.

Patience

In a society of immediate gratification and satisfaction, we are starting to view patience as a nuisance. We now get instant coffee from our Keurig in a matter of seconds. If we send a text and someone doesn't respond within a minute, we think something is wrong. We associate patience with inconvenience. The uncertainty of the future can give us anxiety and frustration. It removes our power and control. Patience involves trusting that our lives are a journey and not just a stop at the amusement park every day.

Creative flow will not be an everyday constant force. You will go through many challenges. Trust the process. Stay the course. Don't bail out after the first taste of adversity or failure. Live in hustle-ville. You can overcome the feelings of doubt by refusing to stand down. Don't quit. Don't sell the mine that you spent so long digging; you could be 3 feet away from the vein of gold.

Do you know the Harry Potter journey through defeat? J.K. Rowling went to 12 different publishers that all turned her down, before finding one that believed in her and agreed to publish the first novel.
https://www.yearon.com/blog/jk-rowling-failure

The Elephant Rope

As a man was passing the elephants, he suddenly stopped, confused by the fact that these huge creatures were being held by only a small rope tied to their front leg. No chains, no cages. It was obvious that the elephants could, at any time, break away from their bonds but for some reason, they did not.

He saw a trainer nearby and asked why these animals just stood there and made no attempt to get away. "Well," trainer said, "when they are very young and much smaller, we use the same size rope to tie them and, at that age, it's enough to hold them. As they grow up, they are conditioned to believe they cannot break away. They believe the rope can still hold them, so they never try to break free."

The man was amazed. These animals could at any time break free from their bonds but because they believed they couldn't, they were stuck right where they were.

Like the elephants, how many of us go through life hanging onto a belief that we cannot do something, simply because we didn't succeed before?
That is part of learning; we should never give up the struggle in life. -Unknown

What About When I Feel Stuck?
Feeling stuck is simply a block. The emotions usually felt are helplessness, lost, depressed or confused. In order to remove the block, you need to remove yourself from the physical space that you are in. It's almost the opposite of a tornado drill. Don't seek cover - get outside. Crank up some jams in your car and go for a drive. Music has a magical power to jump start the good chemicals in our brains. The best goal should be to find a social environment that promotes conversation. Go to a coffee shop and ask a stranger how their day is going. An even better goal is to stimulate your senses by going to a concert or performance. The human connection will inevitably stir up the magic that you thought you lost. The worst thing you could do is lock yourself in your room and binge watch movies. This does nothing for your quest but waste valuable time.

Travel and seek adventurous activities. Experiences outside of our normal 'routine' produce stimulus and memories that generate nostalgia. If you are seeking inspiration, plan a trip.

Engage your passions. Change the world.

6. TRUE SELF

Authenticity means being our true self.

Our Character + Our Values + Our Passions - Ego = Our TRUE SELF

If you haven't already, take time to study the psychology of Ego. Ego is the mask that you hide behind. It is false confidence. It is wanting to dress like her or look like him. Ego is what defines your personality. It has no concept of right or wrong, it only wants to reach pleasure and is associated with being entitled. The ego tricks you to think that the world revolves around you. We give into the bad ego when we compare ourselves to others and create self-doubt. We start to create an unrealistic vision of ourselves. We do need our ego to mediate between our needs and desires and our characteristics and values. To uncover our authentic self, we simply need to get rid of the illusion of who we are. The true self is who we are when no one else is around. When we sing in the shower there is a beautiful realization that there is no one around to judge us. The ego causes you to become defensive when someone criticizes you. The true self recognizes the emotional stimulus from your reaction to fight back, takes a deep breath to calm down and becomes mindful that you are perfect the way you are. If you are at peace with who you are, you will not feel the emotion that other people are your enemies. Ego puts up boundaries but can never protect you. It actually creates a prison. Let love guide your heart. The authentic self lets go of perfectionism and pursues to define characteristics and values of the true mind. Begin to love your wholeness, both good and bad, not your image. Christopher Miller wrote: "Do not submit to self-doubt and do not listen to that voice telling you that you are fat or weak or sensitive." Self-doubt is our biggest enemy.

Ages 16 - 25 are the opportune years to 'develop' character. By this time, we have made enough mistakes to understand the difference between good from bad. The critical parts of the rational brain involved in decision making are typically fully developed around age 25.

Character refers to a set of moral beliefs that define how we treat or behave with others and ourselves. It is the mental and moral traits that are learned behaviors and required by society. We have the ability to develop our own character.

Focus on developing character, not personality. Character is how hard we work out. Personality is what we choose to wear to the gym. Personality is your mask. Personality is your swagger. It is not a requirement of society or success. We will not discuss personality in this book because it does nothing for the greater good. Personality is often linked to vanity which is described as inflated pride in one's appearance.

Character is formed by habits. The previous chapters lay out the foundation for acquiring your traits. For example, people with a high level of fitness tend to be organized, punctual, persistent, accountable and passionate.

Let's start to define your Characteristics -
Take a look at the positive and negative characteristic traits listed below. Use a **BLUE** marker to highlight or circle the traits that you feel you have that you are proud of. Use RED for the traits you have that you wish you didn't. Use GREEN to show the traits that you don't have, but would like to.

Adventurous	Caring	Empathetic	Depressing	Active	Pessimistic
Agreeable	Kind	Fair	Irresponsible	Obnoxious	Disorganized
Brave	Persistent	Fearless	Humble	Bossy	Helpful
Anxious	Cold	Cowardly	Optimistic	Dangerous	Petty
Aggressive	Understanding	Weak	Patient	Thoughtful	Assertive
Openminded	Sensitive	Focused	Likeable	Possessive	Jealous
Immature	Angry	Greedy	Impolite	Shallow	Forgetful
Responsible	Fake	Difficult	Moody	Competitive	Appreciative
Courageous	Intelligent	Funny	Reliable	Cooperative	Frightening
Annoying	Loyal	Mean	Respectful	Sloppy	Witty
Boring	Loving	Disloyal	Peaceful	Flexible	Enthusiastic
Charming	Gullible	Genuine	Energetic	Resilient	Neat
Clever	Polite	Hard Working	People-Pleaser	Creative	Demanding
Hateful	Independent	Arrogant	Sneaky	Careless	Unforgiving
Compassionate	Easy-Going	Crazy	Playful	Friendly	Giving
Considerate	Weird	Picky	Selfish	Irritable	Disrespectful
Lazy	Encouraging	Honest	Dedicated	Judgmental	Indecisive
Cheerful	Athletic	Confident	Wise	Accepting	Mature
Chatty	Quiet				

Virtues are the essence of our character. Select a few that are a true representation of who you are today.

Acceptance	Courage	Forgiveness	Idealism	Passionate	Sincerity
Assertiveness	Creativity	Friendliness	Integrity	Patience	Temperate
Authenticity	Detachment	Generosity	Imaginative	Peace	Tenacious
Beauty	Determination	Gentleness	Joyfulness	Perseverance	Thankfulness
Caring	Dignity	Graciousness	Justice	Preparedness	Tolerance
Cleanliness	Encouragement	Gratitude	Kindness	Purposefulness	Trust
Commitment	Enthusiasm	Harmonious	Love	Reliability	Truthfulness
Compassion	Ethical	Helpfulness	Loyalty	Respect	Understanding
Confidence	Excellence	Honesty	Moderation	Responsibility	Unity
Consideration	Fairness	Honor	Modesty	Reverence	Visionary
Contentment	Faith	Hope	Optimistic	Self-discipline	Wisdom
Cooperation	Flexibility	Humility	Orderliness	Service	Wonder

Start by picking three virtues that best describe you from the list and write them down here.

Virtue   >

Virtue   >

Virtue   >

Now that you understand more about your virtues, you can start to write your personal virtue statements.

Here are some examples:

Love - I am committed to authentic love through compassion, kindness, acceptance, patience, understanding, forgiveness, selflessness and humility. I am committed to bringing forth authentic love by having integrity, honesty, and truthfulness in living into my values.

Compassion - The essence of my coaching is generated from a place of compassion, being genuinely concerned for others by being kind, empathetic, caring, sensitive, patient, humble and understanding.

Authenticity - I am committed to bringing forth my authentic self by being real and honest with myself and others, by owning my vulnerabilities and accepting my humanness. I am open, transparent, vulnerable and courageous in self-disclosing and sharing with others who I am.

Focus on these statements and commit to discerning what your true beliefs are. Once you feel comfortable with them, start to write your Human Potential Statement (Purpose).

Here is an example:

I am committed to constantly bring forth change within myself by striving to be the highest expression of myself. Through my own personal insights, experiences, learnings and understandings, I am committed to teaching others how to become the highest authentic expression of themselves.

Embrace your inner awesomeness and weirdness! That is what makes you authentic. We are all different. We were not born with a product description or neon headline. We are each unique unto ourselves. Do not worry about living up to society's expectations. Please your own inner attention first instead of craving other people's attention. Accept yourself as you are. False-self creates an illusion of hierarchy, as if some people are better or more favored than others. The truth is that everyone and everything is interconnected. Authenticity starts when you accept yourself for who you are, the way you are.

7. SPIRITUAL BALANCE

As you step out the door to live on your own, be sure to pack your spiritual bag. Each one of us walk out of many different home conditions. Some may have very little exposure to a spiritual environment and others may have extreme experience with Godly love. Some may have a family member that is a priest, minister, rabbi, shaman, monk, imam, or other leader and some may have a family member who is an atheist. No matter what door you leave, you will need help along the way. 'I can do this on my own', said the fool who fell down a well in the woods ... alone!

Some of us leave home without the support of family and with low psychological or financial resources. Without guidance or direction, it is easy to become self-absorbed and victimized. Be wary of toxic anxiety that may tend to promote fear, depression, emotional paralysis and various forms of addiction and escapism. If you find yourself in this position, know that you are not alone. Make a decision today to find a mentor that will listen and help answer some of your questions and offer a few solutions for direction. You may have a community leader that would be willing to share some advice or books that could open your mind to a much bigger world than the one you are currently living in.

How do we find direction? Is the path from childhood still the right fit? Should you seek a new community whose worship styles and values are more aligned with your emerging identity? Will you become spiritual but not religious? Will you attend church or go on a walk in the woods to meditate?

Start to look inward. Once you begin to focus on your inner spiritual peace, you will start to understand that your worldly pursuits, success in business and obsession over money will never give you fulfillment. One of the biggest lessons for humans is the revelation that we need connection with others and a trusting relationship with God / Infinite Intelligence /

Creator / Yahweh / Christ / Supreme Being / Elohim / Jehovah / Allah / Almighty / Brahmana / ETC.

Religion should not be confusing, regressive, political or exclusive. There shouldn't be my God, your God, his God, her God or their God. God is Love and Love is Universal. Spirituality is a personal journey that is within your own heart, mind, body and soul. It is the revealing of love in totality. Richard Rohr said "It is the freedom to care for your world and everyone in it. Not political freedom, but the freedom to care for your own needs, without ego. Spiritual awareness is the freedom from yourself."

There are hints of our culture shifting toward an All-Inclusive Religion and Radical Unity. We are slowly moving away from tribal religions and the exclusivity that they promote. The true purpose of spirituality is to access a connection to Infinite Intelligence. It is not claiming a religion or label. Accessing this connection opens new dimensions to a more meaningful life. Instead of pondering about the intricacies of theology, focus on kindness, compassion, selfless service and gratitude.

Spiritual Discipline
The best habit you can begin practicing and include as part of your development plan: refrain from looking at your phone, TV or computer for the first ten minutes you are awake!

Commit to making this your routine. Your mind is clear and has not been influenced by images on social media or the thoughts of your studies or work. Devote this precious time to the following:

> Thoughts of gratitude - for everything in your life
>
> Thoughts of supplication - for your needs and health
>
> Thoughts of intercession - for the needs of others
>
> Ask for the opportunity to serve others with compassion

Ask for spiritual warfare tools to fight evil temptation

Take time for breathing sessions throughout the day. Meditation is a way to center yourself and find a mentally clear and emotionally calm state. The benefits are pretty shocking.

Subscribe to motivational emails or blogs. Below is a list of good books to help you get closer to understanding spiritual paths:

- *The Alchemist* (Paulo Coelho)
- *The Power of Now* (Eckhart Tolle)
- *Being In Balance* (Dr. Wayne Dyer)
- Way of the Peaceful Warrior: A Book That Changes Lives (Dan Millman)
- A Return to Love (Marianne Williamson)
- The Untethered Soul (Michael A. Singer)
- The Four Agreements (Don Miguel Ruiz)
- *The Universal Christ* (Richard Rohr)
- *Tao Te Ching (Stephen Mitchell)*
- *Eat, Pray, Love* (Elizabeth Gilbert)
- The Book of Awakening (Mark Nepo)
- *A Course in Miracles* (Dr. Helen Schucman)
- Start Where You Are: A Guide To Compassionate Living (Pema Chodron)
- The Art of Happiness (Dalai Lama XIV)

Find the place where you feel a spiritual connection and go there often. Some people feel most connected on their quiet back porch. Others enjoy concentrating on prayers while they are driving alone. Some feel most engaged while in the woods camping or fishing. Others feel a high level of spiritual connection while worshiping in church. Some find that place while meditating in a group. Spiritual transcendence means leaving the physical world behind.

If you are struggling with the desire to dive deeper into your spiritual life, try attending a few different churches. You never know if the right fit for you is just one more block away. Check into programs that may be offered during the week such as small groups. Smaller peer settings can offer a greater awareness of spiritual connection and give you a more intimate sense of community. Take pride in the home church that you choose and make sure that you leave feeling encouraged and not beaten down. Kristi Talley once said "I'm proud of our church, I needed it and didn't even know it." Church should be a time to give thanks, honor your beliefs, gain education and experience fellowship in a comfortable setting. Group worship is good for everyone. If you disagree, then you haven't found the right one yet. Keep searching brothers and sisters! By the way, church is a translation of the Greek word ekklesia, which was originally defined as a place where 2 or more people gather together to worship the divine, not a majestic building of architectural design.

Living a more spiritually fulfilling life does not mean you have to quit your job, sell all your belongings and go meditate on a hilltop. Start by recognizing your desire to grow. Take a few moments during the day to read spiritual literature. Formation through practice is essential for your journey. Your beliefs will change over time with your life experiences and education. Intentionally focus on incorporating more spiritual practice and knowledge into your life. Make time for your daily walk and you will soon feel the connection we are all inherently seeking. If you do not make time, disruption will creep in as quickly as the night.

8. RELATIONAL BALANCE

Family

You may have two parents, one parent or no parents! You may not have any family connection at all. You may have been raised in the woods by wolves. *If you have...we need to meet for coffee tomorrow.* Familial status does not have to be defined by blood or a birth certificate. Family of origin refers to the significant caretakers and siblings that a person grows up with. This could be biological or adoptive family.

No matter who your family is, it is almost impossible to argue that you have been influenced by them. Your behaviors, likes, dislikes, environmental preferences and societal influences have all been controlled, influenced or manipulated by them. These are considered your family of origin issues. It is important to recognize what influences or experiences have impacted you and they should be separated into good and bad. Take a day to reflect on this, write them down and then destroy the notes. By doing this, you will start to liberate your mind. Drop the anchors that are keeping you from moving on. Now you are free to focus on your path, without the weight of any past burdens. If you have deeper issues from your childhood, you might need to confront the people who hurt you. Speak with a psychologist or counselor first.

Family should be the circle of people that you trust, love, honor and call on to be there for you when you need it the most. Family should have fun together and be a part of as many life experiences as the universe will allow.

Some people call certain families broken, dysfunctional or absent. This is just another label. Family is family! Every family is different. There are many professions that require parents to travel or be away from home for extended periods of time. Military families are a prime example. Sacrifices are part of life and we should be completely grateful for those people in our lives that make them for us.

One big challenge with family is earning their respect. You should never feel like you have to 'act' older than you are. Others will have high expectations of you. If you think they are always undermining your decisions or treating you like a child, earn their respect! Most times this can be accomplished by showing them that you are making good decisions through respectful communication. If someone thinks you should go to college and become president of a company, then talk to them like you already do. Share your Personal Development Plan and Career Plan. Let them know that you want to move to a far-off city to pursue your dreams of getting a degree. If they truly want you to live a life of fulfillment, they will help you plan the move.

There is a love in this world that is unconditional. As humans, we have learned this concept from infinite wisdom. It can be defined as affection or love without limitations or conditions. Do not let a disagreement of lifestyle or belief come between you and your family. Do not let time slip away from you connecting with them. Make a calendar reminder to call a family member every week at least just to say hello and ask how they are doing. You can respectfully let them know that you had a quick 5-minute break in your day and wanted to check in.

Be sure to set reminders about birthdays. Celebrate holidays together. Be present and avoid distractions when you are with them. Staring at your phone all Thanksgiving Day is annoyingly selfish and disrespectful. If you are on a tight budget around Christmas, get thrifty and creative to come up with gift ideas on the cheap. One cool idea for parents or grandparents that still have boxes of old photographs is to digitize them using the PhotoScan app and save them in Google Photos. Once you have them loaded into cloud albums, you can share with everyone as a gift for collaboration.

Love Partner
We all grow up in unique home environments. Some children are nurtured more than others. Some are disciplined more.

Some are abused, some are praised and some are neglected. For most of us, our childhood experiences are transferred into our adult relationships.

No matter what your situation is or was, you have the opportunity to change your view of and approach to love.

It starts with first loving yourself. Once you and your partner are complete within yourself, you will both come from a place of abundance. It will be a relationship of choice. "I choose to be with you" instead of "I need you to complete my unhappiness or voids within myself." Al Talley wrote "Your happiness will come from within and not from your spouse. Allow each other to be the essence of who you are while enjoying the presence of each other in mysterious and magical ways."

Focus on finding your authentic self before you commit to someone else. Once you have a solid foundation of physical health, mental health, emotional health, convictions, authenticity, purpose and financial health, then you are ready to start looking for a partner.

> Love should be like the ice cream truck. Don't go chasing it around town.
> Patiently wait for it to show up at your house.
> -C.C. Talley

Don't chase love. When it's right, it will come to you.

"If I could go back in time and change anything, what would it be"?
One common answer from adults is the following: I wish I would not have made life altering decisions based on immature lust. Don't fall for the trap. Love relationships are the hardest to sustain.

Here are some great books to check out:
> Things I Wish I'd Known Before We Got Married (Gary Chapman)

All About Love: New Visions (Bell Hooks)
The Five Love Languages (Gary Chapman)
Hold Me Tight (Dr. Sue Johnson)
The All or Nothing Marriage (Eli J. Fenkel)
The Seven Principles for Making Marriage Work
(John N. Gottman and Nan Silver)
Love Sense (Dr. Sue Johnson)
Receiving Love (Dr. Harville Hendrix)

What are the signs that you are meant to be together?

Dating- are you comfortable with how extremely clean or grossly unclean your partner is? Do you know if they have a large debt or a large inheritance? Do you like the way they look first thing in the morning ... with no makeup on and hair in a mess? Will they hold you when you hurt, or will they judge you? Are they truly funny? Do you like the same cultural music and movies?

Unfortunately, there is no complete playbook for love. If you are both coming to the relationship as authentic and whole people, then you should be able to set some shared goals.

Goals for Building a Lasting and Meaningful Love Relationship

Be Vulnerable. Talk about your past and your needs. Earn each other's trust!! Trust is not given away freely. Help each other evolve. Solve problems together. Don't argue for the sake of arguing. Never put each other down or hold the past against them. See the worth and value in each other. Feel privileged to be around each other. Be blessed because you GET to walk through life with your partner. Trust love and commit to romance (pray for strength and reject outside temptation). Practice respectful and daily communication. State clear expectations. Make sure that you are in alignment and agreement before making any big decisions. Affirm support for each other's passions. Be happy for each other's successes. Harbor good thoughts for each other. This is a big one!!! Agree to always make time for intimacy and limit distractions. Tell each other all your deep secrets. Relax and be yourself. You should never feel like you have to perform or be someone else. Accept each other for who you are. Cook for each other. Discuss financial compatibility such as lifestyle desires and values. Is debt a deal breaker? Are you going to be a couple that spends or saves?

Commit to being loyal. Be 100% sure that you both have a mental and heartfelt connection to each other, not just physical attraction. Temptation is everywhere and if you are not completely committed to each other, it will most certainly come knocking. Infidelity (cheating) is the grim reaper of love. Here are two quick suggestions:

1) Avoid - Focused glances at people that could produce irrational thoughts of jealousy.
2) Avoid - Your cell phone. Time together is sacred. Social media and the news can wait. That amazing piece of technology can kill a relationship if it becomes your focus.

Understand the power of your words! Always speak words of kindness. Any demeaning or degrading vocabulary should be locked out of your love world. Avoid speaking to friends or co-workers in a negative manner about your loved one.

Practice active listening. One of our biggest communication problems is that we do not listen to understand, we listen to reply. Active listening can be accomplished by concentrating on what is being said, not just hearing the words coming out, while thinking about how we are going to get our point across when they are finished. Instead of focusing on our own opinions, we should remain non-judgmental and truly listen. Practice feeling empathy while listening.

Welcome each other home with open arms, light candles, dance in the kitchen and go on long walks.

One of the most freeing, uplifting and validating emotions of life is when you realize that your partner believes in you and loves you for all your craziness!

Be sure to choose someone who you can laugh with. Moments of uncontrollable laughter will bring you closer than a fancy dinner in Paris.

Friends and Social Relationships
Social Intelligence means treating others with respect in order to bring out their best. The beautiful chaos of young adulthood will introduce countless people into your life. Be sure to engage in warmhearted relationships with the people that invest their time and energy into you. Focus on the relationships that mean the most to you and have shared values. True friendships should be built on quality instead of quantity.

We should all do our best to avoid negative people. Our youthful years introduce a few toxic situations of social disassociation and disconnect. Have you ever said 'they just don't fit in' or 'I'm not popular enough' or 'nobody likes me.' Where do these feelings come from? They primarily emerge from self-doubt, jealousy, difference of beliefs and competition in sports or academics. The biggest might be competition for love. Recognizing our differences and honoring people for being authentic is an essential part of our growth.

"Our culture has accepted two huge lies. The first is that if you disagree with someone's lifestyle, you must fear or hate them. The second is that to love someone means you agree with everything they believe or do. Both are nonsense. You don't have to compromise convictions to be compassionate."
-Rick Warren

It's OK to be opinionated, just don't become the obnoxiously barking chihuahua in the room.

Ask 'What' instead of 'Why'

When we are faced with adversity, we often ask ourselves: Why did this happen to me? Why are they being so mean? Why can't I get better?

Here is a suggestion. Stop asking 'Why' and replace it with 'What'.

These questions may provide you with better answers: What is causing this discomfort? What pain is causing them to be so mean? What is blocking me from getting better?

Healthy relationships are a vital component to our personal health and wellbeing. Strong relationships can help reduce stress, promote healing, influence best behaviors, provide a greater sense of purpose and even extend life. Choose your friends wisely.

Do not be afraid to love. Learn to forgive. Forgiveness will free you from fear and doubt.

9. OCCUPATIONAL BALANCE

If humans could write the rules of life, we would all know our true calling at an early age and always find happiness in our work. But that is not the case. Recent studies have shown that on average, people entering the workforce will hold fourteen different jobs and two to three different careers. That is a much different path than previous generations that worked one job their entire life in hopes of collecting a pension at the end of their career.

One third of your life is spent at work. The time that you spend working makes a huge impact on the quality of your life. Be purposeful when searching for a professional career. Contrary to what we have heard, knowledge is not power. It is possible power. Knowledge alone will not attract money, unless it is organized through a plan of action. So, what direction should we focus on?

Entering the Workforce or Looking to Transition
There are over 12,000 Career Choices in the U.S.
If you don't know what you are good at or what your interests are, take an aptitude test or career test.
https://www.rasmussen.edu/resources/aptitude-test/
https://www.careeronestop.org/Toolkit/Skills/skills-matcher-questions.aspx

Job seekers once printed resumes on high-quality linen paper that cost a lot of money, slide them into clear cover binders and hand deliver them to the receptionist at the company they were applying to. These days the preferred method for recruiting is LinkedIn and other job search engines like Indeed, CareerBuilder, ZipRecruiter, Glassdoor or Monster. Be sure that you maintain respectful social media accounts. If you submit your LinkedIn profile, know that your Instagram, Twitter and Facebook accounts will more than likely be viewed as well. Spend time researching how to create the best LinkedIn profile and resume that you can. Try to avoid buzzwords. Make sure that your pictures are professional 'looking' and that you are smiling. Determine the top attributes that truly set you apart. Think about your core values. Perhaps they include: Integrity (Always do what is right), Discipline (Own it to the finish), Relationships (Be passionate about what you do and serve others with dignity), Value Creation (create value in everything that you do). What makes you unique? What is your mojo? Create your secret sauce. Sauce like a boss!

Before applying for a job or starting your own business, come up with a list of at least 10 questions that can be answered by someone who has been successful in your potential role, to your satisfaction. Use your LinkedIn network to mine for contacts. Internships are a great opportunity to test ride an industry.

Salary, benefits and commute distance are important details, but there are other questions you should ask before accepting a job. For example, if you want to become a Real Estate agent, ask what the financial requirements are to get into the business. If you think you want to sell Real Estate as a side hustle, make sure you have around $2,000 to get into the business, 60+ hours of time for pre-license education and tons of local contacts to start your hustle.

Find a career that you are passionate about, is aligned with your values and one that will utilize your skill set. You should truly care about the success of the whole business. If you are following in the path of your family, make sure that you are doing it for yourself and not to please them. Have a drive and happiness about your occupation. Do not seek out security or money. No job is secure. Seek happiness.

Learning, Training, Dedication, Persistence

"Nothing in this world can take the place of persistence. Talent will not; nothing is more common than unsuccessful men and women with talent. Genius will not; unrewarded genius is almost a proverb. Education will not; the world is full of educated derelicts. Persistence and determination alone are omnipotent."
-Calvin Coolidge

Be dedicated to learning and training. Once you have built up your skill set, you will have the power to leverage yourself. Talent is not given to us freely at birth. It is cultivated through deliberate practice. Malcolm Gladwell wrote a book called 'Outliers'. He discusses the factors that contribute to high levels of success. One of the big studies that he concluded is it takes 10,000 hours to master something. The best athletes and touring musicians have all surpassed the 10,000 hours of practice and performance. Do you know the story of Bruno Mars? He lived in a maintenance building shack for a few years as a kid and skipped breakfast so that he could pay for lunch while living in LA. He grossed $100,000,000 from touring in 2018. If you want to be the best, you have to be willing to put in the time. Your skills and character are what will propel you toward success, not your education. Don't let your competitors outwork you. Competition is the axis on which our economic world spins

Earning Trust and Respect
Just as in our personal relationships, trust in the business world must be earned. The best way to earn respect is through accountability. If you are late to work or meetings, fail to finish projects on time or finish cleaning your station thoroughly, you will lose trust. Always be early. You respect someone when you respect their time. If you have a problem with timeliness, change your habits. Set an alarm earlier. Plan for bad traffic. Don't stay up so late. Do what you say you will do. Finish the task. Deliver results!

Proper Communication

There is a big generational communication gap that exists in today's world. There are 5 generations currently in the workforce: Traditionalists (born before 1946), Baby Boomers (born 1946-1964), Gen X (born 1965-1976), Gen Y or Millennials (born 1977-1997), and Gen Z (born after 1997). The biggest contribution to the gap has been the advancement of technology and the internet. There has been a paradigm shift in how we communicate. Baby Boomers tell stories of how they use to travel hundreds of miles to a sales meeting that was set as the result of a mailed letter, give a personal presentation to solidify the sale, drive to a pay phone to place the sales order, drive back to the office to speak with the fabrication team and get home at midnight. This process can all be accomplished today over the internet in 5 minutes with email and video conferencing. The advancement in technology has certainly improved productivity but has eliminated a lot of need for human connection. We must protect the elements that are necessary for human advancement. Most importantly, empathy and care.

We have an opportunity to build a dynamic multi-generational workforce. The most respectful question to ask a colleague or client is 'how do you prefer to communicate'? Get on the same page. Some older generations still prefer a phone call over text or email. Here are a few other quick tips:

Always say hello (good morning) and goodbye (goodnight). If you walk past someone on the way into work and fail to acknowledge their existence, you have disgraced them and lost any form of respect.

Practice active listening. Understand what was communicated, process your response through emotional intelligence, then reply. "Most people do not listen with the intent to understand; they listen with the intent to reply." -Stephen R. Covey

Avoid conversation about topics that do not involve your work. Conversations about politics and religion are hot buttons for some people. Practice honorable workplace behavior. Check your bags of dirty laundry at the door.

Communicate consistently. Don't shut down because someone didn't have the reaction to your idea that you expected them to have. Be sure to share your ideas. You have a voice and should be heard. Your opinions matter.

Body language is very important in the workplace too. You have the ability to communicate things without saying one single word. When you shrug your shoulders, you say "I don't know." When you raise your eyebrows, you say "Excuse me? Did I hear you correctly?" When you avert your eyes, you are saying "I'm not that interested" or "I have other things on my mind." Your body language in an interview or performance review can either promote you into the position you are seeking or demote you to the exit door. Make sure that you are conveying confidence by maintaining eye contact, not fidgeting your hands or feet and sitting or standing with a good posture at a comfortable distance.

Success in the Business World
Greatness and success should be defined by you, not a narcissistic business partner or manager. It starts with your goals. Are your goals to serve others? What is success and how do you measure it? Is it a personal feeling of accomplishment or is it recognition by your peers? Grant Cardone talks about the 10x Rule. He states that by setting goals that are 10 times what you think you can achieve and taking massive action that is 10 times the effort of everyone else, you will receive 10 times the results. The take away from this idea is that we need to set goals that are almost unobtainable. This will help keep your drive alive.

"A bad attitude is like a flat tire, you can't go anywhere until you change it." -unknown

Every day, you control your attitude, effort, behavior and actions. Hold your values high and don't give into negative pressure. Be known as the leader of integrity!

Find a Mentor or Coach
A mentor or business coach might be a critical piece to your success puzzle. Start by asking the leadership team at your current company if they could recommend someone. If you are a startup business owner, reach out to the local SCORE (Service Corps of Retired Executives) office and be sure to read 'The Lean Startup' by Eric Ries. You might be able to find a trusted advisor on LinkedIn. What activities do you need help with? Is it financial acumen or organization? They will certainly be able to help you build your personal brand. Look for more than just one coach. Build your own team of Shark Tank judges. Be sure to have your questions ready before you meet with them. They will want to see that you are ready to work super hard. When you finish this book, please check out the Personal Coaching tab on our website. I would love to help you work on all areas of life balance, accomplishing your goals, overcoming your fears and achieving fulfillment.

Write a Career Plan
Here is a spreadsheet to get you started. Edit this template to fit your role. Be sure to log onto www.achievingfulfillment.com/book-tools and click the link to access the Google Sheet version. Save your own copy first and then you will be able to edit for your own development plan.

WHO I AM	VALUES	COMPETENCIES	
CURRENT COMPANY:		Sales	
POSITION:		Marketing	
CURRENT SKILLS, KNOWLEDGE, EXPERIENCE:		General Management	
		Communication	
		Strategic Planning	
		Budgeting	
		Project Management	
		Organization	
		Leadership	

GOALS	12 MONTHS	2 - 5 YEARS	LONG TERM
POSITION / ROLE / TITLE			
WHAT SKILLS DO I NEED TO DEVELOP			
WHAT DO I NEED TO LEARN / CERTIFICATE / DEGREE			
WHAT RESOURCES WILL I NEED			
HOW WILL I MEASURE SUCCESS			
TARGET DATE FOR REVIEW			

Start your career by creating the tools that you need to become successful. Some helpful aids might include customer relationship management software (CRM), daily task lists, analytics, operational checklists, organization charts, support contacts. Hold yourself accountable. Develop a healthy obsession for accomplishing goals. There will be sacrifices that you have to make. Just make sure that they are made for the greater good, not just for your personal pleasure.

Quality of Work:
Uphold Integrity in every product or service that you deliver. Do not settle for good or just OK. Give your best effort and deliver greatness to every single customer. If you burn the bun, throw it away. If the shortcut will negatively affect your client or patient in the long run, do not move forward with the option. If it takes a little longer to perfect, let the customer know that you are not comfortable delivering an inferior or incomplete product.

Leadership v Management:
We lead people! We manage zoos! That doesn't quite explain the difference between the two words but it is close. Leadership is more than being the smartest person in the room or the person with the most experience. A leader moves people to do their best work. A leader unifies everyone with shared goals and values. Effective leaders lead through inspiration, not intimidation.

"Extreme Leaders cultivate love, generate energy, inspire audacity and provide proof" -Steve Farber (Radical Leap)

If you are seeking a career in management or starting your own business, take time to study Authentic Leadership. Here are a few notes of wisdom: Always remind staff that you are available and want to 'listen'. Lead by example. Practice servant leadership. Clarify your expectations. Create transparency. Show loyalty. Praise positive behavior.

Unfortunately, there will be times when you need to manage bad attitudes. The challenge is in responding with education and not reacting with anger. This is one of the greatest tests of emotional intelligence. Practice leading, training and guiding with compassion and care. Conflict resolution should become one of your top skills. Like anything that is worth learning, it is difficult at first, but the more experience that you gain, the easier it becomes. Become a master of words (not eloquence but appropriateness). At the end of the day, your team only wants to know that you care for them.

Always celebrate with the people that helped you succeed, not just a select few that you think deserve praise. Everyone! The custodian is just as much a part of the team as the lead surgeon. Many people have left employers due to a lack of recognition. Often, when they leave, they become the previous company's new competition.

Work Life Balance
Managing our workload can be very overwhelming at times. Sometimes it may be necessary to pull an all-nighter, but if you work 100 hours each week, you may suffer in other areas. Set boundaries early in your career and protect them. If you are on your phone all night instead of spending quality time with your sweetheart, you may be waking up alone. Always be aware of time. It can slip away quickly. Take pride in your work. Honor yourself. Find the balance.

10. FINANCIAL BALANCE

Did you have a lemonade stand or sell anything at the street as a kid? What did you do with your profits? Did you buy new roller skates or invest half of it in a retirement account and spend the rest on a gift for your parents as a thank you for helping out as the financial backer?

Instilling healthy financial habits was probably not at the top of our parent's priorities. Can you remember them having a conversation with you about building a budget, designing investment goals, filing taxes or setting up a retirement account? Luckily, it's never too late to start a financial plan. We all come from different social and economic backgrounds. Do not let that define you.

There is a financial epidemic in our country called 'Living Paycheck to Paycheck'. If that epidemic has one bad month, the recipient could end up broke, homeless and soulfully bankrupt. Without a plan, healthy habits and dedication, any one of us could end up there. Doubt + Debt = Depression = Death of mind, body and spirit.

Let's set a goal to increase your financial awareness and develop a plan for managing your money. Education is the key to your financial independence. There is not a 'one size fits all' model but with a little more knowledge, you will better understand where you need to focus your current goals. Here are three great resources:
Smart About Money
https://www.smartaboutmoney.org/
Dave Ramsey
https://www.daveramsey.com/store/youth
Chris Smith
https://iamnetworthy.com/

Set up an Emergency Fund
Start with $1,000 as a first goal. Make sure the money is liquid (immediately available) in a checking or money market account with a debit card. Only allow yourself to use this for unexpected medical expenses, expenses if you lose your job or source of income, urgent home or car repairs or family emergencies. Set a goal for having it secured in 12 months. If you are purchasing a house, increase the balance to $3,000.
Do not use this account for shopping, vacations, holiday gifts, student loans or starting a business.

Personal Budget
This is an itemized list of all your expected income and expenses. Great businesses reconcile their income and expenses daily. Treat your life like a great business. You should plan on managing this at least on a weekly basis. A good spreadsheet can replace the old checkbook reconciliation method. This will allow you to track your habits and plan for how your money will be spent and saved. Mint app is great for tracking in real time if you connect it to your bank account.

Here is a spreadsheet to get you started. Be sure to log onto www.achievingfulfillment.com/book-tools and click the link to access the Google Sheet version. Save your own copy first and then you will be able to edit for your own personal budget.

Income	Frequency	Amount	Monthly	Yearly
Income #1	Monthly	$0	$0	$0
Income #2	Monthly	$0	$0	$0
Additional Income	Monthly	$0	$0	$0
Total Budgeted Income			$0	$0
Expenses	Frequency	Amount	Monthly	Yearly
Housing				
Mortgage/Rent	Monthly	$0	$0	$0
Maintenance	Yearly	$0	$0	$0
HOA Dues	Yearly	$0	$0	$0
Total			$0	$0
Transportation				
Car loan #1	Monthly	$0	$0	$0
Car loan #2	Yearly	$0	$0	$0
Gas	Monthly	$0	$0	$0
DMV Fees	Yearly	$0	$0	$0
Parking Fees	Yearly	$0	$0	$0
Oil Changes	Yearly	$0	$0	$0
Repairs	Yearly	$0	$0	$0
Maintenance	Yearly	$0	$0	$0
Total			$0	$0
Medical				
Office Visits	Yearly	$0	$0	$0
Dental	Yearly	$0	$0	$0
Glasses/Contacts	Yearly	$0	$0	$0
Specialty Care	Yearly	$0	$0	$0
Medications	Yearly	$0	$0	$0
Medical Devices	Yearly	$0	$0	$0
Total			$0	$0
Utilities				
Natural Gas	Monthly	$0	$0	$0
Electric	Monthly	$0	$0	$0
Water	Monthly	$0	$0	$0
Sewer	Monthly	$0	$0	$0
Trash/Recycling	Monthly	$0	$0	$0
Phone (home)	Yearly	$0	$0	$0
Phone (cell)	Monthly	$0	$0	$0
Internet	Monthly	$0	$0	$0
Cable	Monthly	$0	$0	$0
Total			$0	$0
Personal				
Clothing	Yearly	$0	$0	$0
Gym Membership	Yearly	$0	$0	$0
Hair Cuts	Yearly	$0	$0	$0
Baby Sitters	Yearly	$0	$0	$0
Child Support	Yearly	$0	$0	$0

Category	Frequency			
Alimony	Yearly	$0	$0	$0
Total			$0	$0
Entertainment				
Subscriptions	Yearly	$0	$0	$0
Eating Out	Monthly	$0	$0	$0
Vacation Fund	Monthly	$0	$0	$0
Total			$0	$0
Household Items				
Groceries	Monthly	$0	$0	$0
Toiletries	Monthly	$0	$0	$0
Total			$0	$0
Giving				
Tithing	Yearly	$0	$0	$0
Charities	Yearly	$0	$0	$0
Christmas Fund	Monthly	$0	$0	$0
Birthday Fund	Monthly	$0	$0	$0
Wedding/Anniversary Fund	Monthly	$0	$0	$0
Total			$0	$0
Pets				
Vet Visits	Yearly	$0	$0	$0
Food	Monthly	$0	$0	$0
Medicine	Yearly	$0	$0	$0
Total			$0	$0
Insurance				
Homeowners Insurance	Yearly	$0	$0	$0
Renters Insurance	Yearly	$0	$0	$0
Health Insurance	Monthly	$0	$0	$0
Auto Insurance	Monthly	$0	$0	$0
Life Insurance	Yearly	$0	$0	$0
Disability Insurance	Yearly	$0	$0	$0
LTC Insurance (long term care)	Yearly	$0	$0	$0
Total			$0	$0
Taxes				
Real Estate Taxes	Yearly	$0	$0	$0
Personal Property Taxes	Yearly	$0	$0	$0
Total			$0	$0
Debt Reduction				
Credit Cards	Yearly	$0	$0	$0
Personal Loans	Yearly	$0	$0	$0
Student Loans	Monthly	$0	$0	$0
Total			$0	$0
Education				
Tuition	Yearly	$0	$0	$0
Children's College Fund	Monthly	$0	$0	$0

School Supplies	Yearly	$0	$0	$0
Total			$0	$0
Savings				
Emergency Fund	Monthly	$0	$0	$0
Misc savings	Monthly	$0	$0	$0
Total			$0	$0
Total Budgeted Expenses			$0	$0
Difference			$0	$0

Spending

Stick to your budget. Understand needs vs. wants. Needs are essential for you to live and work. Wants provide comfort for fun or leisure. You can definitely live without wants. Until you have your emergency, investment and retirement accounts satisfied, do not give into spending money for wants. Practice the art of frugality. Frugal does not mean cheap! Living a frugal life means being responsible until you are able to produce an income that can accommodate more wants. The less money you spend, the less money you need. The hard truth is that young adults do not deserve everything. You should earn what you desire. Learn to be happy with what you have and definitely do not spend money trying to impress someone. Believe in delayed gratification. If you delay the gratification of spending money and focus on saving, you will build wealth and become prosperous sooner. Here is the secret: Spend Less, Save More.

Delayed Gratification

"In the 1960s, a Stanford professor named Walter Mischel began conducting a series of important psychological studies. During his experiments, Mischel and his team tested hundreds of children — most of them around the ages of 4 and 5 years old — and revealed what is now believed to be one of the most important characteristics for success in health, work, and life. Let's talk about what happened and, more importantly, how you can use it.

The Marshmallow Experiment

The experiment began by bringing each child into a private room, sitting them down in a chair, and placing a marshmallow on the table in front of them. At this point, the researcher offered a deal to the child. The researcher told the child that he was going to leave the room and that if the child did not eat the marshmallow while he was away, then they would be rewarded with a second marshmallow. However, if the child decided to eat the first one before the researcher came back, then they would not get a second marshmallow. So, the choice was simple: one treat right now or two treats later. The researcher left the room for 15 minutes.

As you can imagine, the footage of the children waiting alone in the room was rather entertaining. Some kids jumped up and ate the first marshmallow as soon as the researcher closed the door. Others wiggled and bounced and scooted in their chairs as they tried to restrain themselves, but eventually gave in to temptation a few minutes later. And finally, a few of the children did manage to wait the entire time. Published in 1972, this popular study became known as The Marshmallow Experiment, but it wasn't the treat that made it famous. The interesting part came years later. As the years rolled on and the children grew up, the researchers conducted follow up studies and tracked each child's progress in a number of areas. What they found was surprising. The children who were willing to delay gratification and waited to receive the second marshmallow ended up having higher SAT scores, lower levels of substance abuse, lower likelihood of obesity, better responses to stress, better social skills as reported by their parents, and generally better scores in a range of other life measures. The researchers followed each child for more than 40 years and over and over again, the group who waited patiently for the second marshmallow succeed in whatever capacity they were measuring. In other words, this series of experiments proved that the ability to delay gratification was critical for success in life.

And if you look around, you'll see this playing out everywhere. If you delay the gratification of watching television and get your homework done now, then you'll learn more and get better grades. If you delay the gratification of buying desserts and chips at the store, then you'll eat healthier when you get home. If you delay the gratification of finishing your workout early and put in a few more reps, then you'll be stronger. Success usually comes down to choosing the pain of discipline over the ease of distraction. And that's exactly what delayed gratification is all about." (Clear, 2018)

Investments
Albert Einstein once noted that the most powerful force in the universe is the principle of compounding (earning interest on top of interest).

The Rule of 72 in investing builds wealth and is a simple way to determine how long an investment will take to double, given a fixed annual rate of interest. By dividing 72 by the annual rate of return, investors obtain a rough estimate of how many years it will take for the initial investment to duplicate itself. Commit to learning more about these topics. There are various ways to buy and sell investments: mutual funds, exchange-traded funds (ETFs), stocks, bonds, certificates of deposit (CDs), real estate and commodities. If you are not interested in studying about finances but expect to make money, try shifting your thinking.

Big Boi (Antwan Patton) from Outkast wrote:
"I balled throughout my twenties, by thirty, see *I was stashing*, First hundred-thousand, I bought a Lexus
First million, I was twenty, I learned my lesson, I bought some land,
Operation Grind and Stack."

Start your own operation grind and stack
Here is the best way for young adults to get into the game. Start with *Stash* app.
Use this sign up link and start your account -
https://get.stashinvest.com/chriszzojy

Set an auto draft so you don't think about it. Start with $5 each week. Whenever your deposit hits your account, log in and direct your investments. You can also set up a Roth IRA for retirement. You can even set up a regular bank account with debit card for daily transactional needs. Stash has some fantastic educational articles that can further assist you in finding the best path for your investment plan.

Retirement Account
Have you thought about when you would like to retire? What will the golden years look like to you? Will you devote your time to charity work? Will you travel the world? Will you sit on public or private boards and coach other companies? Many employers offer an IRA and will match your annual contribution. This is free (...not really, you worked for it) money towards your retirement. If you are self-employed, you will need to set up a Roth account. Stash app has a great product for this.
See where you stand at your current age and potential investment period by using this investment calculator: https://www.daveramsey.com/smartvestor/investment-calculator

Savings Account
You have the ability to set up more than one savings account. First determine what is most important to you. A vacation fund is an important one. How about one for family health needs or gifts?

Here is a story about a chef that learned a good lesson. He complained about never being able to go on vacation because he was broke and worked every day of the week. He spent $40 going out every night and $6 on vape/cigarettes. When he finally had enough of the same old routine, he asked for help. With a mentor, he determined that he spent $322 each week on things that were detrimental to his health and development. He was depressed and overworked. He agreed right then to make changes for a better life and future. The next day he opened a savings account and quit smoking. He committed to putting half of his going out money into the account every week. He also decided to only go out a few nights and spend the rest of the nights exercising and reading. He asked his manager for 2 nights off each week. Not only did the manager grant him the 2 nights off, but also gave him a raise. The chef booked a trip to Mexico after just 12 weeks. By making a few life altering decisions and creating new healthy habits, he was able to save $1,680 for the vacation.

Credit Cards

Using a credit card is an important step in building healthy credit history. Be sure that you understand credit and the potential for abuse if not used with a plan. Choose a card that fits your needs. Study the terms and features associated with the account. Practice responsible credit behavior by making on-time payments, paying your balance in full, avoid over spending, keep a low utilization rate, check your monthly statements for accuracy, keep your credit card secure and do not request a cash advance (they carry high fees).

Transportation

What forms of transportation do you have available and what do they cost? What option will save you the most money? Will Uber or Lyft save you money? Is an Electric Car an option (be sure to measure your mileage needs and charging station options for functionality). Some people are able to bike everywhere while others have no choice but to use a personal car. If you live on a farm or use your vehicle for towing of course you will need to have that awesome GMC truck. The costs involved in owning a car are on the rise (taxes, insurance, fuel, parking). Public transportation is a low-cost option that allows passengers to text while riding and have peer to peer connectivity. Take time to write out all of your options and the costs associated with each. Decide on the best option that will save you the most money. Whatever you decide, make sure it is safe.

Housing and Real Estate

Are you currently renting or do you own? Renting is making someone else money. Owning is building your own personal wealth. Real Estate is a superior investment. It is an appreciating asset that can be leveraged and has positive cash flow. Could you imagine generating $100,000 a year from rental income, pretty much just by managing your properties and finding tenants all the while building equity that can one day be sold for cash? Compared to investors who rely on the stock market to accumulate assets for their retirement, real estate investments take a different approach. If you accumulate $2,800,000 in income-producing real estate it will pay $50,000 a year in income and continue to appreciate in value over the years, not only covering you indefinitely but also leaving you something to pass on to your children or family. Here's the interesting part, it only takes $700,000 in investment capital to accumulate $2,800,000 in real estate assets. By comparison, it takes about $900,000 in stock investments to achieve a $50,000 per year annual income, assuming that during the 30 years of investing, both types of investments yield a 4 percent return.
Source: (ExpertProperties.com)

Robert Kiyosaki wrote a great book called 'Cashflow Quadrant". He basically states that there are 4 ways to produce income: employee, self-employed, business owner or investor. Becoming an investor will ultimately provide you with the maximum amount of free time and money.

Management is the key to prosperity. Create your **Personal Financial Statement** today and start managing your money. There are a few millionaires that are basically broke because they never figured out how to do this.

Here is a spreadsheet to get you started. Be sure to log onto www.achievingfulfillment.com/book-tools and click the link to access the Google Sheet version. Save your own copy first and then you will be able to edit for your own development plan.

CURRENT ESTIMATED NET WORTH		YEARLY GOALS	
Assets	$0.00	Retirement Account	$0.00
Real Estate Estimated Value	$0.00	Emergency Account	$0.00
Vehicles	$0.00	Investment Account	$0.00
Savings Accounts	$0.00	Car Principal	$0.00
Stocks/Bonds/Mutual Funds/ETF's	$0.00	House Down Pmt	$0.00
Total Short Term Savings	$0.00	Donations / Tithing	$0.00
Other Assets	$0.00	Vacation Account	$0.00
Other Assets	$0.00	Credit Card Debt	$0.00
Other Assets	$0.00	Gifts	$0.00
Total Assets	$0.00	5 YEAR GOALS	
Liabilities			$0.00
Mortgage Loan Balances	$0.00		$0.00
Vehicle Loan Balance	$0.00		$0.00
Student Loan Balance	$0.00		$0.00
Credit Card Balance	$0.00		$0.00
Personal Loan Balance	$0.00		$0.00
Medical Debt	$0.00	LONG TERM GOALS	
Other Liabilities	$0.00		$0.00
Other Liabilities	$0.00		$0.00
Other Liabilities	$0.00		$0.00
Total Liabilities	$0.00		$0.00
NET WORTH	$0.00		$0.00

Wealth is a Perception

What is the definition of wealth to you? Is it a collection of 'stuff' or is it a life of 'minimalism'? It could be perfect health, love in your life, greater financial supply, more friends or the ability to express yourself through use of your gifts. Western society tends to embrace that wealth is the accumulation of money and tangible prizes or things. Many eastern societies acknowledge wealth as a life with minimal personal objects or belongings and includes great relationships with family and connection to the community. The value they bring to the world creates the perception of wealth.

Whatever your vision is, make sure that it is a healthy one. Be sure not to compare your situation with others. Set yourself up to obtain all your goals by managing your finances now.

11. PURPOSE / SERVING

"The things you do for yourself are gone when you are gone, but what you do for others remains as your legacy." - Unknown

Serving others is the key to achieving prosperity and fulfillment. There it is! Isn't that simple? It almost sounds too easy. This life is not about how high you can climb. It's about helping and serving other people and giving your skills to help aid the betterment of society. Once you decide to start adding value to other people's lives by being of service and living selflessly, you will start to receive in abundance. Help others awaken to their greatest self. You get what you give!

"We make a living by what we get, but we make a life by what we give."
-Winston Churchill

"No one has ever become poor by giving."
-Anne Frank

"Giving is not just about making a donation. It is about making a difference."
-Kathy Calvin

"We rise by lifting others."
-Robert Ingersoll

"Only by giving are you able to receive more than you already have."
-Jim Rohn

"When you learn, teach. When you get, give."
-Maya Angelou

"It's not how much we give, but how much love we put into giving."
-Mother Teresa

"Giving is the master key to success, in all applications of human life."
-Bryant McGill

"At the end it's not about what you have or even what you've accomplished. It's about who you've lifted up, who you've made better. It's about what you've given back." -Denzel Washington

"If you have much, give of your wealth; if you have little, give of your heart."
-Proverb

This statement is very important: Every connection matters!

I once had a restaurant staff that met every Thanksgiving Day to prepare meals, load them in a caravan and pass out downtown to people in need. The meals were not just PB&J sandwiches. We made smoked turkey breast sandwiches with seared Ritz cracker stuffing, lingonberry coulis and thyme aioli on a locally baked bun. Included in the bag were sides of sweet potato soufflé, roasted Brussels sprouts and bacon, and pasta salad. This meal at the restaurant would have easily cost $25. Since these people did not have a Thanksgiving table or family to join, we took it to them and served it with a hug and grateful conversation.

Searching for opportunities to help others
This takes practice but is easy to achieve. Your head was built to swivel and your eyes were designed with peripheral vision capabilities, unless you have a physical impairment. Keep your head on the swivel and your eyes on the prize. You may have just walked past someone that was having thoughts of depression and needed a kind word or hug. There might be a child in your community that will only be able to eat one meal today due to low income. There is a lost soul that is a day away from becoming homeless. There is someone that will be abused tonight because they are too afraid to fight for themselves. Find these people in need and help them!!

One of the toughest challenges to overcome when beginning a life of service is the fear that something bad is going to happen to us if we become vulnerable. Judgement is the enemy! If we become fearful about helping someone because of the way they look, talk, walk or smell, then we have failed before we even started.

Everyone Has a Story in Life
A 24 year old boy looking out from the train's window shouted... "Dad, look the trees are going behind!"
Dad smiled and a young couple sitting nearby, looked at the 24 year old's childish behavior with pity, suddenly he again exclaimed...
"Dad, look the clouds are running with us!"
The couple couldn't resist and said to the old man...
"Why don't you take your son to a good doctor?" The old man smiled and said..."I did and we are just coming from the hospital, my son was blind from birth, he just got his eyes today."
Every single person on the planet has a story. Don't judge people before you truly know them, the truth might surprise you.
Source : https://www.livin3.com/5-motivational-and-inspiring-short-stories

There is a sensation of happiness that is bigger than the one you received opening presents as a child on Christmas. There is a feeling of enlightenment that you can receive from giving. When you become empathetic instead of apathetic, you start to tap into this sensation. Empathy comes from showing or feeling interest, enthusiasm or concern for others. Watch this video and you will begin to experience this feeling.

Transformation for a marginalized neighbor / not your average makeover:
https://www.youtube.com/watch?v=ogKxFY6W_MY&t=59s

Empathy and dignity establish the roots for altruism and the philanthropic spirit. Stewardship gives us a sense of belonging and responsibility to our community. Community can mean street, neighborhood, city, county, state, country, other countries or global issues. We were created to help, love and show kindness to one another. You have gifts that the world needs. Use them! Help people release the feeling of victimization and pain. Make a difference. Change lives. Become obsessed with serving others.

Here are some great philanthropic stories about love and hope that you should check out:

-Hero's with Aprons Instead of Capes
The Story of Ryan Hidinger and Jen Hidinger-Kendrick
https://thegivingkitchen.org/who-we-are

-Providing Opportunity and Hope
The Story of Brian Preston and Lamon Luther
https://www.lamonluther.com/pages/our-story

Have you ever asked yourself if you will ever fully achieve success or significance?

"Success is when I add value to myself. Significance is when I add value to others." -John C. Maxwell

Here are a few lists of some amazing charities.

NON PROFIT DIRECTORY SEARCH	100 LARGEST US CHARITIES
NATIONAL	
Feeding America	National Alliance on Mental Illness
Humane Society of the United States	Habitat for Humanity
The Breast Cancer Research Foundation	Boys & Girls Clubs of America
Hope for the Warriors	American Cancer Society
Scholarship America	American Red Cross
The Alzheimer's Assosciation	American Heart Association
Lukemia & Lymphoma Society	Polaris Project
Prevent Child Abuse America	Make A Wish Foundation
National Alliance to End Homelessness	Wounded Warrior Project
Mental Health America	Disabled American Veterans
Boot Campaign	American Humane
Autumn Years	Susan G Komen
Prostate Cancer Foundation	St. Jude Children's Research Hospital
GLOBAL	
United Way Worldwide	Stop the Traffik
Unicef USA	Task Force for Global Health
Operation USA	Salvation Army
Global Fund for Women	Direct Relief
Charity: water	Goodwill Industries International

Food for the Poor	Compassion International
Samaritan's Purse	The Nature Conservancy
MAP International	Save The Children
Americare Foundation	World Wildlife Fund

Start your own list of serving opportunities that are close to your heart:

	ORGANIZATION	CONTACT	PHONE	EVENT
NEIGHBORHOOD				
CITY				
NATIONAL				
INTERNATIONAL				

12. RECEIVING

"Giving opens the way for receiving."
-Florence Scovel Shinn

Life is meant to be lived joyfully. Don't pursue the idea of happiness, but instead, pursue a lifestyle that results in joy. Happiness is your team winning the title or getting a promotion at work. Your job will not provide fulfillment. Pleasure, wealth, honor and dignity will not give you joy. They are all good, but not enough. Since everything is interconnected, it is a natural consequence that if you give, you must receive. We need to train our hearts to be open to receive the gifts of the world. Self-love, human connection and dignified relationships provide joy. That is the fulfillment and prosperity that we are all seeking.

Sometimes a gift is of value to us, but other times it is not. The connection is what is most important. When you receive a gift, be sure to acknowledge it, look the giver in the eyes with a smile, say thank you and feel a warmth in your heart for their presence in your life. Your actions and words should say "I see you and am thankful for you." Never reject a gift no matter how big or small. It could be as silly as a rock or as monumental as a house. When you grab that rock, your reaction should be the same as when you grab the key to the house. Your emotions may be different but your reaction should be consistent. Embrace the joy of the moment and the opportunity to dive deeper into the relationship.

If you were fortunate enough to go to camp when you were young, then you surely felt this joy. Do you remember leaving feeling like you were floating on a cloud because of all the new friendships and connections that you made? That is called the 'camp-high' feeling. You were able to participate in activities with complete strangers and make lifelong memories. Adults can still achieve this immense level of love. Tony Robbins hosts seminars where 2,500 people gather for a week and leave completely transformed by the compassion that they felt and connections that they made.

Part of receiving is opening our senses to enjoy the hard work of others through art, music, performance and other forms of entertainment. There is a great story that was posted in the Washington Post by Gene Weingarten, titled 'Pearls Before Breakfast'. The story graciously points out how easy it is to miss one of the best musicians in the world, playing some of the finest music ever written, with one of the most expensive instruments ever made. That is pretty embarrassing when you think about it. Be sure to stop and listen to street corner musicians. Go to concerts, plays, orchestras, local art shows, museums, dance performances. Watch the band play at halftime.

Another undeniable gift that we must receive is the amazing beauty of our world. Be adventurous. Travel! The saddest stories are ones of people who never leave their hometown. Routine in our lives is good but stagnation is bad. Being stagnant can cause the feeling of boredom or even depression. It comes from seeing the same environment every single day and in the same order. Traveling outside of our hometowns allows us to experience new cultures and gain a respect for the diversity of civilizations. Get cultured! These days, you can be thrifty with traveling. Airbnb and VRBO offer great rates and more privacy than a hotel. Do some research and come up with a list of 10 destinations that you would like to visit in the US and 3 international destinations. Create a list of vacations and the year that you want to take the trip. Be sure that this list is connected to your Travel Savings Account and budget.

Keep a mind of gratitude, not a scorecard.
Be sure not to keep score when it comes to giving and receiving. People usually give what they can. If you have someone in your life who seems to never 'give back', just keep giving. You may not ever receive anything back from them, but you will get it from another person in your life.

"We must face, confront, and grow beyond the archaic belief that we are allotted just so much good, and when we use it up, we are bereft. The universe is showering blessings to us constantly, and we receive as much as we let in. The mind is the gateway to all blessings. The key to receiving a generous supply is to give it."
-Alan Cohen

13. CONCLUSION

Personal Development Plan

Start your plan today! We are required to take action and change our behaviors in order to advance our development. This will allow us to realize our true potential. Here is a template that you can use. Take all the information that you wrote down earlier and plug into this document.

Be sure to log onto www.achievingfulfillment.com/book-tools Click the link to the Google Sheet version. Save your own copy first and then you will be able to edit it for your own development plan.

Personal Development Plan									
Year									
Virtues	1								
	2								
	3								
	4								
Top Passions	1								
	2								
	3								
	4								
Human Potential Statement	*								
		Body	Mind	Spirit	Finance	Work	Family	Social	Serving
Strength									
Weakness									
Threats									
Goals									
		AP	Teacher	Mentor	Coach	Mentor	Focus	Focus	Mentor

Name								
MINI GOALS	Body	Mind	Spirit	Finance	Work	Family	Social	Serving
January								
February								
March								
April								
May								
June								
July								
August								
September								
October								
November								
December								
Financial Statement								

Time Management and Organization

Balancing a personal schedule can be a difficult task, but it should be simple if you put in the time to develop a fortified system. Effective calendar management starts with finding a system that works best for you. Start with a spreadsheet or pen and paper. Make an outline and spend time managing the activities and connections in your life that matter most. Your ability to choose between important and unimportant will bring you the greatest success. Discipline yourself to choose the most healthy and productive opportunities and activities. If something important is not scheduled in your calendar, distractions will certainly take its place. How many times each day are we distracted by shiny things? Instead of bouncing all over the place with squirrel-like behavior, develop the focus of a cheetah hunting prey.

Here is a tool that everyone can use. Be sure to log onto www.achievingfulfillment.com/book-toolss Click the link to the Google Sheet version. Save your own copy first and then you will be able to edit it for your own development plan.

CREATE YOUR OWN EFFECTIVE WEEKLY SCHEDULE

SCHEDULE FOR THE WEEK OF
_____

TIME	MONDAY	TUESDAY	WEDNESDAY	THURSDAY	FRIDAY	SATURDAY	SUNDAY
6:00 AM	Exercise	Exercise	Exercise	Exercise	Exercise		
6:30	Water Garden	Water Garden	Water Garden	Water Garden	Water Garden		
7:00	Shower	Shower	Shower	Shower	Shower		
7:30	Breakfast	Breakfast	Breakfast	Breakfast	Breakfast		
8:00	Pareto Time	Pareto Time	Pareto Time	Pareto Time	Creative		
8:30	>	>	>	>	>		
9:00	>	>	>	>	>		
9:30	>	>	>	>	>		
10:00	Email	Email	Email	Email	Email		
10:30	>	>	>	>	>		
11:00	Pareto Time	Pareto Time	Creative	Pareto Time	>		
11:30	>	>	>	>	>		
Noon	Lunch	Lunch	>	Lunch	Pareto Time		

12:30 PM	Centering	Centering	Lunch	Centering	>		
1:00	>	>	>	>	Lunch / Planning		
1:30	>	>	>	>	>		
2:00	>	>	>	>	Filing		
2:30	>	>	>	>	Data Entry		
3:00	>	>	>	>	Email Cleanup		
3:30	>	>	>	>	>		
4:00	Email	Email	Email	Email	Email		
4:30	>	>	>	>	>		
5:00	>	>	>	>	>		
5:30	>	>	>	>	>		
6:00	Yoga	Dinner	Dinner	TRX Class			
6:30							
7:00	Dinner		Band Practice	Dinner	Friends Dinner		
7:30	Call Relatives			Call Relatives			
8:00							
8:30							
9:00							
9:30			Prayer				
10:00	Meditation	Meditation	Go To Bed	Meditation	Meditation		
10:30	Prayer	Prayer		Prayer	Prayer		
11:00	Go To Bed	Go To Bed		Go To Bed	Go To Bed		

FREE TIME - time to rest, relax and rejuvenate	
CREATIVE TIME - time to generate new ideas or study	
PARETO TIME - deliver the product/service that is core to your work	
SUPPORT TIME - administrative functions necessary to support you	

Pareto Time is the 80/20 rule. It states that 20% of your activities, customers, products or tasks will account for 80% of your results, sales, profits or value of what you do. This means that if you have a list of ten items to do, two of those items will turn out to be worth as much or more than the other eight items put together.

The next step is to find one app or calendar that will be your main source of daily organization.

Keeping Good Notes
Google Keep and Evernote are great apps to help collect all the information that is coming at you. Some people have a challenge remembering names. If you fall into this category, use one of these apps to record the contact's name, an association that you relate to them (Dave needs a shave) and even a picture of them. Some people use imagery as a shortcut to associate the information that we want to remember. For example, you can imagine a pirate with a wooden leg for a woman named Peggy or a big grizzly bear for a man named Harry. A good cognition system will help you keep track of all the balls that you are trying to juggle.

Abraham Maslow said, "Either step forward into growth or step back into safety."
Be dedicated to implementing what you have learned.

Here is your Treasure Map and Magic Secrets:

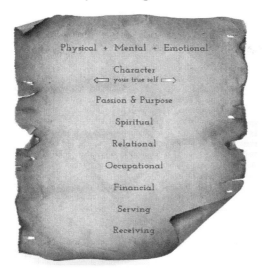

Physical + Mental + Emotional

Character
⟵ your true self ⟶

Passion & Purpose

Spiritual

Relational

Occupational

Financial

Serving

Receiving

Start every day with a great attitude and disposition (view of yourself and of the world)

Take the Stairs. Stay away from Angry Bears

Choose Love and Hope over Fear and Doubt

Find and Protect Your Ultimate Courage

Be Confident In Your Decisions and Efforts (confidence means 'to trust')

Create Healthy Habits by Choosing Good Discipline and Organization

Uncover your Passions and Purpose

Balance All Areas of Your Life

Focus on Goodness

Always look for Opportunities to Serve Others

Be present to receive the gifts and grace that you are given

Laugh Uncontrollably

Life is all about the journey. Watch sunrises ignite, waves crash, clouds roll, sunsets melt, and fireworks burst under moonlight. Be good to yourself. Help others. Improve the world. Enjoy the ride!

NEXT STEPS

Log on to our website and sign up to enjoy additional tools and benefits. New opportunities are currently being developed.

http://www.achievingfulfillment.com

Personal coaching sessions (see below)

Store

Local networking connections

Volunteer at team events

Ticket offers to local shows

No AdWords, just motivation, education and tools

PERSONAL COACHING

Our goal is to help individuals create personal development plans that inspire lasting results.

FULL COMPASS™
360 degree approach to coaching

Review lifestyle management, behavioral change and character development

Assess strengths and opportunities for skill development

Dream and create a vision

Prioritize and select areas of immediate focus

Establish personal development goals

Create a new schedule

Monitor progress

R. I. S. K. AWARDS

We support a community of positive change and acts of goodness. As a result, we have created the:

Recognition of Success and Kindness Awards

We encourage you to tag us in your social media posts that depict images and stories of your personal success or acts of service and grace toward others. Our goal is to select the best submissions annually and document the stories with our production team. Please be sure to use:

#achievingfulfillment

REFERENCES / LINKS

Morin, Amy (March, 2017) *13 Things Mentally Strong People Don't Do: Take Back Your Power, Embrace Change, Face Your Fears, and Train Your Brain for Happiness and Success*

Millman, Dan (1998) *Everyday Enlightenment: The Twelve Gateways to Personal Growth*

Bonnie, Richard; Sepúlveda, Martín (Dec 2014) *Health Affairs: Investing In The Health And Well-Being Of Young Adults*
https://www.healthaffairs.org/do/10.1377/hblog20141215.043313/full/

Clear, James (2018) Behavioral Psychology, Willpower*: 40 Years of Stanford Research Found That People With This One Quality Are More Likely to Succeed*
https://jamesclear.com/delayed-gratification

Maslow's Hierarchy of Needs
https://www.youtube.com/watch?v=O-4ithG_07Q&feature=youtu.be

Eating Right
https://www.eatright.org/food/nutrition/dietary-guidelines-and-myplate/eating-right-isnt-complicated

Check out these 42 raised garden bed plans:
https://morningchores.com/raised-garden-bed-plans/

Foods that cause inflammation:
https://www.medicalnewstoday.com/articles/320233.php

Total Body Stretching Warm-Up
https://www.youtube.com/watch?v=sTxC3J3gQEU

10 Perfect Morning Stretches to Increase Energy for Women

https://www.youtube.com/watch?v=eOWJsw_ARB0

Here are some cardio workouts that you can do at home or in the park: https://www.verywellfit.com/best-home-cardio-exercises-1231273
24 minute cardio for Women
https://www.self.com/story/a-sweaty-24-minute-cardio-workout-you-can-do-in-your-living-room

Cardio for men
https://www.mensjournal.com/health-fitness/5-home-cardio-workouts-fat-loss/bear-crawl-finisher-workout/

13 Things Mentally Strong People Don't Do
https://www.inc.com/amy-morin/13-things-mentally-strong-people-dont-do.html?cid=search

10 Reasons Why Real Estate is a Superior Investments
https://www.expertprops.com/ten-reasons-why-real-estate-is-a-superior-investment/

The Power of Compounding Interest
https://www.thebalance.com/the-power-of-compound-interest-358054

Check out 'The Fallacy of Work / Life Balance'
https://www.youtube.com/watch?v=hJIkgFn2efc
(9:06 if we are free to not be perfect.....)

US News 100 best jobs
https://money.usnews.com/careers/best-jobs/rankings/the-100-best-jobs#best-job-ranking-1

NOTES

NOTES

NOTES

NOTES

71398258R00062

Made in the USA
Columbia, SC
26 August 2019